High-Performance Medical Libraries

High-Performance Medical Libraries

Advances in Information Management for the Virtual Era

Edited by Naomi C. Broering

Meckler

Westport • London • Melbourne

Library of Congress Cataloging-in-Publication Data

High-Performance medical libraries : advances in information
    management for the virtual era / edited by Naomi C. Broering.
       p. cm.
    Includes bibliographical references and index.
    ISBN 0-88736-878-6 : $
    1. Medical libraries--Automation. I. Broering, Naomi C.
Z675.M4H47 1993
026.61'0285--dc20   93-11527
                                                      CIP

British Library Cataloguing-in-Publication Data is available.

ISBN 0-88736-878-6

Meckler Publishing, the publishing division of Meckler Corporation,
    11 Ferry Lane West, Westport, CT 06880.
Meckler Ltd., Artillery House, Artillery Row, London SW1P 1RT, U.K.

Printed on acid free paper.
Printed and bound in the United States of America.

CONTENTS

v

INTRODUCTION

Dreamers, visionaries, and researchers contribute greatly to the progress of mankind. They are the progressives that create new knowledge and push our frontiers far beyond what the typical person can imagine. These pioneers exist in many professions, and the medical library world is especially fortunate to have its share of such enlightened individuals. Medical libraries also benefit greatly from advances made by the National Library of Medicine (NLM).

In the initial planning and preparation of *High-Performance Medical Libraries*, we decided the case studies included in the book should bring together some of the most advanced thinking and trends in medical libraries. We wanted to set the stage internationally for the next generation of virtual medical libraries by compiling a group of cases on innovative and unique projects. We chose projects that we believe will have enduring and critical impact on the profession. And, we chose authors highly recognized for their outstanding contributions on technology in libraries.

In keeping with the "high performance" theme, the chapters in this book cover key areas of concern that should not be overlooked. Certainly, the NLM's efforts in developing the Integrated Advanced Medical Information Systems and the work leading toward the High-Performance Computing and Communications Act are critical for the emergence of virtual medical libraries. Also under the auspices of the NLM we included papers on the Unified Medical Language System™ (UMLS®) and the Semantic Network.

The impact of technology is witnessed most clearly in the birth of networks, electronic resource sharing, document delivery, and full-text systems. Now that many of our libraries have integrated library systems, we are prepared for the next logical step which is to venture beyond the online catalog to develop extended systems and databases, manage information such as human genome systems, and create image workstations that can deliver slides, illustrations, photographs, and such to our users when they search the online catalog.

It is important to include advances in corporate, hospital, society, and public libraries in a book of this nature. Here the contributing authors provide a broad and universal perspective that extends the breadth and scope of the readings. This section is designed for librarians at varying levels of technology implementation.

Lastly, but immensely critical, is the section on computer training laboratories and medical education software. It is in demonstration labs and media training centers where library users learn about the latest software and how to use computers. The evolution of these centers and the services and research they perform is becoming an accepted responsibility of high-performance medical libraries. The essential role of the NLM is especially important for librarians interested in promoting use of educational software at their institutions.

In compiling these readings, we encouraged the authors to write the way they felt most comfortable. In other words, they could portray their accounts freely, pointing out positive and negative factors they deemed important to discuss. Several chapters emerged from papers presented at the Computers in Libraries 1992 annual conference held in Washington, D.C. Some of the projects were partially funded from sources other than the institutions' budgets. In that respect, we are indebted to the NLM.

We feel the case studies gathered in this work provide interesting and instructive stories of future directions in the medical library arena. It is hoped the book is educational and useful to librarians planning to implement advanced information technology.

Naomi C. Broering

CHAPTER 1.
FROM IAIMS TO HIGH-PERFORMANCE
VIRTUAL LIBRARIES AND MEDICAL
INFORMATION MANAGEMENT

Naomi C. Broering
Director, Biomedical Information Resources Center
and Medical Center Librarian
Georgetown University Medical Center
Dahlgren Memorial Library

Abstract

The National Library of Medicine's (NLM) initiative to implement the Inte-
grated Advanced Information Management System (IAIMS) in 1982 has played
a major role in enhancing medical libraries. Because the concept of IAIMS is
to integrate and improve the flow of information in a medical center, it has
placed the medical libraries in a focal position for the transmission of medical
information. This chapter traces the NLM's intent in supporting the IAIMS
grant program and historical events leading to this successful and popular
program. Highlights listing the institutions participating in IAIMS, recent
changes in the program, and the potential role of IAIMS in the High-
Performance Computing and Communications System are discussed.

Introduction

The Integrated Advanced Information Management System
(IAIMS) program was, and is, the right thing to do. It has been a
significant initiative and notable success in developing organization
mechanisms to manage the knowledge of medicine. It has placed
health science institutions in the forefront of information systems
integration and communications networking. Results to date are
starting to have a positive and observable impact on research, patient
care, and education. . . . IAIMS institutions are models for further-
ing the spread of planning, designing, and managing large-scale,
institution-wide integrated information networking programs.[1]

Donald A.B. Lindberg

1

This chapter traces the IAIMS program through a decade of growth and highlights evolutionary milestones leading to the newest IAIMS effort, the creation of the high-performance computing and communications initiative, and the emergence of virtual medical libraries for the future. These advances are destined to transform our work and daily lives, how we seek and handle information, how we acquire knowledge, and how we make new intellectual discoveries.

IAIMS was an extremely visionary program because it established a solid foundation for the work which will be accomplished in the next decade. Academic medical centers needed to organize medical information before networking could be accomplished. Medical libraries needed to implement integrated systems and become major players in their institution's information network system. The vision needed seed funding to develop models, to test the concepts, and to demonstrate the range of possibilities. The story of how a small program made such an impact, as to change the way medical centers manage information, is highlighted below.

Background

In 1980, the National Library of Medicine (NLM) funded an Association of American Medical Colleges (AAMC) study on the impact of new information technologies on the role of health sciences libraries. The resulting report, published in 1982, described the need for integrated information management systems at academic health sciences centers that would bring together scholarly records, medical data systems, library information systems, and research systems.[2] The report included recommended actions which the NLM and other health institutions including medical libraries should undertake. In response to the recommendations, the NLM launched a long-range IAIMS program to fund competitive strategic planning projects at four institutions. The original four institutions were Columbia University, the University of Maryland, the University of Utah, and Georgetown University.

In 1984, a symposium held at the NLM covered the progress, plans, and experiences of these institutions. In welcoming the first symposium attendees, Dr. Donald A.B. Lindberg, director of the NLM, noted the achievements of medical informatics today and "what information systems and humans can do synergistically"[3] that was not possible twenty years ago. Approximately 150 individuals from seventy-two academic medical centers attended the program. The symposium proceedings provided valuable background on IAIMS as well as the initial reports from the participating institutions.[4]

Interest in IAIMS continued to grow. In 1984, NLM expanded the IAIMS prototype program by announcing a three-phased grant applications structure: Phase I, planning; Phase II, model development; and Phase III, implementation.

A second symposium held by NLM in March 1986 also was well attended. By this time, there were eight universities that reported their progress on IAIMS—the original four and four new institutions—Johns Hopkins University, Baylor University College of Medicine, Duke University, and the University of Cincinnati. In addition, leaders in medical informatics discussed changes affecting medical education. The effort of each medical center was shaped by what occurred before IAIMS, by the institution's own character, and by its ability to address needs.[5]

On the surface, the model projects appeared to be quite different. Yet, despite surface differences, there were many common elements. Each institution needed to upgrade what might be termed basic "infrastructure" or "core resources" that would support the model project in the NLM grant as well as other projects. Specifically, each institution needed a network, the capability to train or educate its users, and general purpose software, hardware, and facilities. Considerable technical support to enable users to acquire information access skills was an essential component of the IAIMS infrastructure that the institutions needed to address. Institutional software and technical systems were also enhanced. The IAIMS sites expanded their databases and information resources, so they could extend services to users. Organizational and behavioral issues loomed equally large. There was and still is concern about policies and protocols for security and access to institutional online systems.

Generally, the institutions enhanced library services by incorporating automated access to information systems in their IAIMS projects. The library is an important component in each plan and its electronic databases are viewed as essential. The libraries have undergone subtle, but important changes, emerging as information centers for their institution. Their responsibilities include more than just books, journals, and audiovisuals; they now include in-house databases and information resources in a variety of automated formats.

NLM Funding for Medical Information Management

Generally, Phase I (planning) awards were nearly $250,000 for two years. Phase II (model development) projects were awarded for three years at around $400,000 per year. Phase III (implementation) awards were approximately $750,000 per year for five years. Recently, the NLM reported that seventy applications of the various phases have been reviewed for funding. Of these, thirty-one awards have been made to seventeen institutions and five are currently in Phase III. Although NLM has been able to fund few institutions, the basic goals of the IAIMS initiative have been achieved.[6] A number of institutions are examining the role of information technology, several are investing their own resources to develop systems and networks, and considerable resource sharing among institutions is taking place. Table 1 lists the seventeen institutions who were operating IAIMS projects in 1991. Funding for Yale University occurred in 1992 which brings the total to eighteen institutions.

What began as a program primarily to improve medical information management at academic health sciences centers was broadened slightly. IAIMS projects were supported at one professional association, the American College of Obstetrics and Gynecologists, and one hospital, Rhode Island Hospital.

In 1992, the program was changed and renamed the Integrated Advanced Information Management System (used to be called the Integrated Academic Information Management System)—still using the IAIMS acronym. The NLM funding cycle is now divided into two stages: Phase I (planning, up to two years of funding at a maximum of $150,000 per year) and Phase II (implementation, $500,000 per year for five years).[7]

Implementation of an IAIMS is an exceedingly expensive undertaking. Because there is such a need to cope effectively with medical information

TABLE 1. IAIMS Awards Made Through Fiscal Year 1991

	Phase I Planning	Phase II Modeling	Phase III Implementing
Columbia University, New York, NY	+	+	+
Georgetown University, Washington, DC	+	+	+
University of Maryland, Baltimore, MD	+	+	
Baylor College of Medicine, Houston, TX	+	+	+
University of Cincinnati, Cincinnati, OH	+	+	
Duke University, Durham, NC		+	+
University of Utah, Salt Lake City, UT	+	+	
American College of Obstetricians and Gynecologists, Washington, DC	+	+	
Johns Hokpins University, Baltimore, MD	+		
University of Pittsburgh, Pittsburgh, PA	+	+*	
Dartmouth University, Hanover, NH	+		
Harvard University, Boston, MA	+		
University of Michigan, Ann Arbor, MI	+	+*	
Rhode Island Hospital, Providence, RI	+		
Oregon Health Sciences University, Portland, OR	+	(active contract)	
University of Washington, Seattle, WA	+		
Tufts University, Boston, MA	+		

* Partially funded

Source: Lindberg. DAB: IAIMS: An Overview

management, each medical center is, of necessity, committing significant institutional resources. Furthermore, most of them have secured donations of equipment from vendors. The schools recognize that vast changes must occur in their organizations and that, most of all, IAIMS needs ongoing commitment at all levels in order to succeed.

Today, the IAIMS concept of functional integration and synthesis of clinical, bibliographic, and knowledge-based systems has been accepted as one of the major challenges in medical informatics. This is happening because the rapid growth of medical information and knowledge has made medical decision making immensely complex. It is essential that decision support systems be implemented to help physicians acquire the information they need for patient care and research from the immense body of medical knowledge.[8,9] The pioneering institutions have paved the way, and today there are models to follow.

The future of IAIMS involves growth at all levels of activity because the power of computers and communications systems are more broadly accepted and implemented in the health field. In addition, the electronic patient record has captured national interest. Progress in this arena will impact the IAIMS goal of linking to a variety of information resources to improve patient care. Biomedical researchers especially those working in molecular biology and genetics, are optimizing their laboratory efforts by using computers and networks. Several IAIMS sites have responded to these demands by implementing molecular biology resources and databases in their projects.

High-Performance Computing and Communications

The impact of the High-Performance Computing and Communications Act (HPCC) and the National Research and Education Network (NREN) has not been felt, but the relationship of these important initiatives to IAIMS is apparent and clear. Just as IAIMS enhanced information flow at medical centers, the HPCC Act introduced by Albert Gore, at the time a senator from Tennessee and now vice president, will enhance the information infrastructure of the nation.[10] We are witnessing important changes as this initiative unfolds because the importance of the health field and the role of libraries has become more critical and more apparent. The NLM is the leading biomedical institution involved in planning the HPCC. Dr. Donald A.B. Lindberg, director of the NLM, was recently appointed director of the National Coordination Office for the HPCC interagency program activities.[11]

The HPCC initiative will enhance the ability to rapidly transmit immense amounts of information including images over the Internet and the proposed NREN. In addition, the ability to compute and process complex data to support medical research and patient care will fill a national need, and it is expected that the IAIMS institutions will be heavily involved in HPCC programs.

Emerging Virtual Libraries

Medical libraries, especially those at IAIMS sites, are evolving into virtual libraries with electronic access to large digital files and information resources. As libraries begin to transform collections into digital format and full-text plus images become electronically accessible, a network superstructure will become a vital lifeline linking the library's intellectual and knowledge resources to the health professional. This is, of course, especially important in medicine where time is often so critical.

The role of virtual medical libraries will be magnified greatly as they further the HPCC effort to bring health information to every home, medical center, and school. In the future, virtual medical libraries can be expected to make phenomenal strides in enhancing the country's intellectual productivity and the research, patient care, and education activities they support. The drama lies in how the emerging technologies will be adapted, how the nation's information infrastructure emanates, and how the use of these marvelous resources unfolds during the next decade.

References

1. D.A.B. Lindberg, R. T. West, and M. Corn, " IAIMS: an overview from the National Library of Medicine," *Bulletin of the Medical Library Association* 80 (July 1992): 244–46.
2. N. W. Matheson and J.A.D. Cooper, "Academic information in the academic health sciences center: roles for the library in information management, *Journal of Medical Education* 57 (October 1982): 2.
3. D.A.B. Lindberg, Welcome. Planning for IAIMS. *Proceedings of a Symposium Sponsored by the National Library of Medicine*, October 17, 1984, Bethesda, MD, p. 3.
4. D.A.B. Lindberg, Foreword. *Proceedings of a Symposium Sponsored by the National Library of Medicine*, October 17, 1984, Bethesda, MD, p. v.
5. Introduction, IAIMS and Health Sciences Education, *Proceedings of a Symposium Sponsored by the National Library of Medicine*, March 12, 1986, Bethesda, MD, pp. 1–2.
6. Lindberg, West, and Corn, 244–46.
7. NIH Guide, August 1992.
8. N. C. Broering and H. E. Bagdoyan, "The impact of IAIMS at Georgetown: strategies to outcomes," *Bulletin of the Medical Library Association* 80 (July 1992): 263–75.
9. N. C. Broering, "Fulfilling the promise: implementing IAIMS at Georgetown University," *Medical Progress through Technology* (1993). In press.
10. 102nd U.S. Congress. High-Performance Computing Act of 1991. (Public Law 102–194, December 9, 1991.)
11. "Members in the news," *Bulletin of the Medical Library Association* 81 (January 1993). In press.

Chapter 2.
IAIMS at Georgetown University: The Emergence of a High-Performance "Virtual Library"

Naomi C. Broering
Director, Biomedical Information Resources Center
and Medical Center Librarian
Georgetown University Medical Center
Dahlgren Memorial Library

Abstract

The Integrated Advanced Information Management System (IAIMS) project as it has unfolded at the Georgetown University Medical Center is examined in this chapter. Georgetown has undergone all three phases of IAIMS: planning, model development, and implementation (currently ongoing). In addition, the IAIMS-related research and corporate equipment grants have provided funds to extend the project even further. The vital role of the Medical Center Library and its emergence as a "virtual library" of the future are traced during the past ten years. Critical highlights include the Library's development of the Knowledge Network of Databases, Scholar Workstations, the Biomedical Information Resources Center for teaching, System Integration, and Resource Sharing. The Knowledge Network databases are comprised of bibliographic, information, diagnostic, and molecular biology systems. Design of educational software including an electronic textbook, history and physical writer, and digital slide libraries are discussed as they pertain to the IAIMS concept.

Introduction

The goal of the Integrated Advanced Information Management System (IAIMS) at Georgetown is to provide effective access to information essential for clinical decision making and patient care management. Effective access can be achieved if a broad range of biomedical information is made available at the place where it is needed, when it is needed, for example, in the health practitioner's office and at the patient's bedside. Such information can come from multiple sources, in many formats: it can include patient laboratory test results, X-rays, patient demographic data, information on drug interactions, library materials from journals and texts, databases on treatment protocols and outcomes, and software programs for clinical diagnosis.

A truly integrated academic information management system would address these key issues. However, because academic medical centers are so complex, they require a coordinated strategic planning effort to create an effective information management system. The National Library of Medicine (NLM) provided such an opportunity through its IAIMS initiative.

Phase I: Medical Center-Wide Planning

In September 1983, Georgetown University Medical Center (GUMC) was selected by NLM to conduct a strategic planning study leading to an institution-wide IAIMS. During the planning, which took two years, GUMC engaged in three major activities: (1) a strategic planning process for IAIMS; (2) an institution self-study, including an environmental forecast; and (3) a ten-year implementation plan.

The aim was to develop an IAIMS plan that would improve information flow by linking the Medical Center in an electronic network of distributed systems. A number of planning activities involving the entire Medical Center were undertaken to accomplish the IAIMS objectives and related tasks. Planning leadership included top-down and bottom-up participation by sixty to seventy individuals from each of the units of the Medical Center (the deans of the Schools of Medicine, Dentistry, and Nursing; the medical director; hospital administrator; and the Medical Center librarian). The librarian assumed the role of principal investigator for the project. Two committees were assigned: the IAIMS planning committee and an executive advisory board.

The outcome was a timely strategic plan to improve academic information management and the transfer of biomedical information through an IAIMS, and to create a Center of excellence and prototype IAIMS to serve as a national resource for other interested academic health sciences centers.

Although planning details are in the university's published IAIMS report,[1] a few pertinent highlights are presented here. The implementation includes: (1) a pilot phase (one to three years); (2) an interim phase (three to five years); and (3) a full/long-range phase (five to ten years). Major IAIMS issues addressed in the plan were: heterogeneous and distributed computer systems, a telecommunications system and local area network (LAN), project operations within the Medical Center infrastructure, financial requirements, leadership, and an evaluation mechanism. The strategy was to test and evaluate all projects before fully implementing them. An initial step was to link sophisticated systems such as the Library Information System (LIS) and the Hospital Information System (HIS) in a LAN. Participating departments and units were to be added in a logical progression beginning with a "clustering" or "mini" IAIMS approach. The Library was to provide core support services, including training in computer use, information resource materials and consulting services. At the hub of these services are the existing LIS, including the mini-MEDLINE SYSTEM™ (a user-friendly bibliographic search system based on NLM's MEDLINE) and other information knowledge databases.[2]

Phase II: The Model Development Project

The three-year model IAIMS grant, awarded by NLM in September 1985, was an umbrella award to provide seed funds for the pilot phase. Georgetown also contributed resources to this cost-sharing effort. The project aims were to create a start-up IAIMS model and begin practical use of applications to be replicated throughout the Medical Center. In the initial years, Georgetown concentrated on supporting changes in health professional education and clinical care, primarily the movement was from memorization and paper learning to teaching problem-solving skills in patient care.

The global approach of the project included five objectives, involving all the Medical Center units, and the initial steps necessary for an IAIMS network system. The objectives were to:

1. establish a communications network system—LAN;
2. develop a neurosciences model to automate the Department of Neurology and link it to the LAN to access the library and hospital information systems;
3. enhance clinical problem solving at all levels of health education by implementing diagnostic systems for the School of Medicine, NEMAS, a teaching program, for the School of Nursing, and expanding the dental titles in miniMEDLINE;[3,4]
4. enhance communications by providing electronic transmission capability and office automation tools such as e-mail, bulletin board, database management, and statistical systems; and
5. provide training and education in the use of electronic resources in an academic information management center.

The BIRC

Once developed, the academic information management center was named the Biomedical Information Resource Center (BIRC). The BIRC was established in 1986 as a facility to provide user training in information access skills and to support the basic educational components of the three schools. Some of the resources for the information center were partially in place in the library. They included a small but well-equipped training laboratory, a collection of software programs, hardware connections to a LAN, and trained personnel to assist users. This facility underwent considerable expansion and renovation. The outcome was a 5,000 square foot center with numerous (over seventy) scholar workstations, two classrooms for instruction on use of computers and access to the IAIMS network, and a laboratory to develop educational software and provide technical assistance.

Core Support Services

Generally, the model development project included core services that required ongoing support such as the LAN, training and consulting services provided by the information center, and electronic transmission of health and management information. Even the special applications that use unique software for unique purposes, such as the model neurosciences experiment and the educational clinical problem-solving modules, required continued support.

Involving the entire Medical Center in the project assured continued momentum and enthusiasm for IAIMS. The intent was to make information from various sources readily accessible to users in the hospital, library, office, laboratory, or at their homes.

Linking Georgetown's Technical Resources

Technically, the projects required an advanced communications system with interface software to link the Medical Center's heterogeneous systems. The Georgetown IAIMS project used the AT&T ISN, which is the campus-wide system and provided links to the Sytek network system used by the hospital. The communications system was a key element in developing the backbone for the IAIMS Knowledge Network. The architectural design was to serve the campus for the long term. Access to shared databases through IAIMS was organized and designed carefully so it could be implemented in a modular approach (see Figure 1).

The Equipment Grants

Georgetown received generous equipment grants from corporations to operate the core support services for the model IAIMS project. These start-up grants came from AT&T, Apple Computer, and Digital Equipment Corporation.

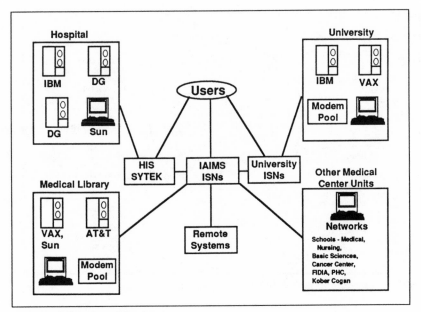

Figure 1. Network architecture

Research Grant To Interface Health Sciences Databases

To put a major IAIMS program in place, Georgetown needed to provide access to basic resources and support tools. An IAIMS research-related grant was received from the NLM to support a study on the feasibility of implementing multiple databases to be accessed through the network. This was accomplished by extending the library's health sciences databases that would be shared and available to users.

Generally, there were four types of health databases identified that handle medical knowledge—five, if management databases are included. They are patient care, research, information/education, bibliographic, and management. Highlighted in Figure 2 under the major categories are the key components of these databases. The research project began with the library, the primary source of recorded knowledge through its bibliographic databases.

The research project determined the degree of database integration needed to help physicians and students. This project focused on the needs of the Lombardi Cancer Center and examined the usefulness of interfacing specialized bibliographic and information databases already in existence. The library used two bibliographic database systems developed at Georgetown (mini-MEDLINE and a similar user-friendly version of Cancer Literature) and two acquired information databases (Physicians Data Query and the MicroMedex

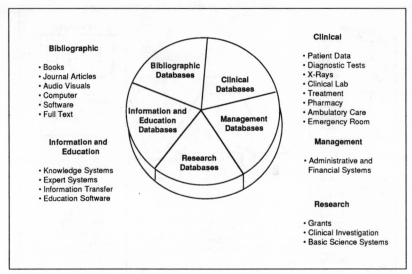

Figure 2. Key components of health sciences databases

Drug Information System). By designing easy-to-use features, the databases were interfaced so users could conduct multiple database searching without rekeying search terms (see Figure 3).

BioSYNTHESIS

Developed in 1987 as part of the research-related project, BioSYN-THESIS was made available to users at the Dahlgren Memorial Library in

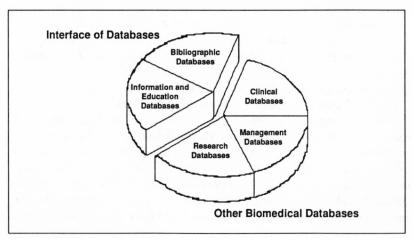

Figure 3. IAIMS research project

1988. It allowed users to search the IAIMS Knowledge Network databases consisting of bibliographic, information, diagnostic, and communications systems. Generally, BioSYNTHESIS is a front-end system which retrieves information stored in disparate databases and computer systems. The system, currently in use at Georgetown, enables users to access various types of information more easily through a single point of entry. Integration of disparate systems functioning on different types of computers has required a staged approach to development of front-end software and a sophisticated solution to system incompatibilities. Because of these complexities, design of BioSYNTHESIS was originally divided into two phases: BioSYNTHESIS I, a gateway system which provides transparent access to selected databases; and BioSYNTHESIS II, an expanded, complex system designed to function as an information finder. BioSYNTHESIS II has changed considerably; it is now a larger integrated system with additional databases, enhanced capabilities, and additional network features. A new phase BioSYNTHESIS III, has evolved because the system and the project have grown in size and complexity. Systems external to IAIMS such as George and GRATEFUL MED are accessed automatically through the BioSYNTHESIS front-end software. This means users can bypass dial-up and logon protocols to look up holdings in the other campus libraries or to search external systems. The Georgetown IAIMS Knowledge Network provides dial-out capability to other non-Georgetown systems and also provides dial-up access from remote sites. The Knowledge Network is heavily involved in the use of Internet, BITNET, and other networks.

As indicated above, BioSYNTHESIS provides a direct connection from a user's terminal to any of the target databases selected for searching. Users can select the databases they wish to search and conduct the search routines for appropriate retrieval. There is a multiple database searching routine that allows users to "highlight text" on the screen, for example a title or medical term, and transfer it to a search in one of three bibliographic databases, the online catalog, miniMEDLINE or ALERTS®/Current Contents™.[5]

Phase III: Full IAIMS Implementation

In 1989, the Medical Center Library received a five-year grant award from the NLM to conduct the IAIMS Phase III (implementation) project. This phase will operate until 1994. The Georgetown vision for this ongoing IAIMS grant project is to create an evolutionary "biomedical world brain" of information resources needed for clinical decision making and patient care management. The major goal of Phase III is to create a Biotechnology and Biomedical Knowledge Network consisting of core information resources that serve as a "decision support system" for education, research, and patient care programs of the Medical Center. The purpose of the Knowledge Network is to implement a family of information databases over five years (1989–1994) that can be accessed electronically by medical center users from home, office, laboratory, or clinical settings. The objectives are to develop sources of knowledge, to establish scholar workstations, to achieve system integration through a LAN and BioSYNTHESIS, to provide computer training in the BIRC, and to implement cooperative projects with other institutions.

The Knowledge Network includes several bibliographic, informational and clinical databases, a variety of scholar workstations, instruction on use of computers, a campus-wide network with LAN nodes and a modular approach to systems integration. The network architecture uses a distributed systems approach, bringing information together via computers, communications, and database systems. Again, because the IAIMS Phase III project is spearheaded by the Medical Library, it has enabled all the medical campus users to benefit directly from new, dynamic services. To develop the Knowledge Network, information resources have been organized into a manageable body of IAIMS databases and systems which are shown in Figure 4. A detailed description of each database is covered in Chapter 9.

The Georgetown approach to develop the Biotechnology and Biomedical Knowledge Network in a modular fashion and to implement selected biotechnology and biomedical databases that are universally useful to campus users has been effective.[6] The focus of the Knowledge Network has been to develop a medical decision support system that emphasizes academic information commonly useful to students and faculty. What began as a Knowledge Net-

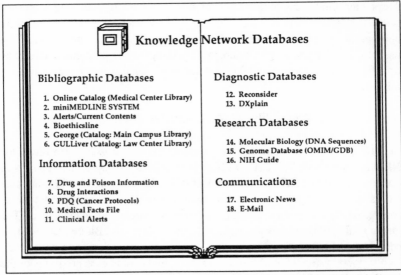

Knowledge Network Databases

Bibliographic Databases

1. Online Catalog (Medical Center Library)
2. miniMEDLINE SYSTEM
3. Alerts/Current Contents
4. Bioethicsline
5. George (Catalog: Main Campus Library)
6. GULLiver (Catalog: Law Center Library)

Information Databases

7. Drug and Poison Information
8. Drug Interactions
9. PDQ (Cancer Protocols)
10. Medical Facts File
11. Clinical Alerts

Diagnostic Databases

12. Reconsider
13. DXplain

Research Databases

14. Molecular Biology (DNA Sequences)
15. Genome Database (OMIM/GDB)
16. NIH Guide

Communications

17. Electronic News
18. E-Mail

Figure 4. Dahlgren Memorial Library Knowledge Network: LIS and IAIMS databases

work with six databases has grown to nearly twenty databases. The organizational grouping of the system was vital because it provided the basis for a logical search mechanism to facilitate user access. Shown in Figure 5, is the icon-based interface to the system. Once a user selects the category to inquire, the next display opens a choice of databases that can be searched in that category (see Figures 6 and 7). The textual interface illustrated in Chapter 9 also uses the same organizational approach. Users find this easy to use and helpful in navigating from one database to the other.

The project provides free access to multiple resources, provides core support services, seeds IAIMS components based in various units and departments, and teaches users how to access the Knowledge Network for their daily work. Business and hospital functions such as financial, patient billing, medical records, and practice plans are not the responsibility of the Georgetown IAIMS. They are maintained by their appropriate units. Special "high-tech" medical technology and research projects in the Medical Center also reside in their unique departments. Most notable of these are the IMACS project in the radiology department and the molecular biology, protein sequence, and digital imaging projects of the NBRF in the physiology and biophysics department.

Scholar Workstations

The scholar workstations are the primary access point to various databases and the means by which users can develop their personal files, conduct special functions, and manipulate information retrieved or stored in the Knowledge Network. Practitioner, student, faculty, and researcher workstations provide user access points to the systems in the Knowledge Network. These workstations vary in power and capabilities depending on the needs of the user. Typically, they store local files, maintain dedicated information and software systems, and have access to the network's databases.

The Practitioner Workstations. This project involves extending the IAIMS model project based in the neurology department and linking their workstations to the HIS clinical lab and X-ray modules to retrieve report results online. The neurology workstations are an AT&T 3B2/400 computer system networked to nine terminals or PCs in physicians' offices throughout the department. These practitioner workstations allow physicians to maintain their own patient records locally, to use the data to monitor treatment, and to conduct clinical investigations.[7] The neurology system has become a model for projects being launched in ophthalmology and psychiatry. Slightly different because of special needs, is the patient database system developed in emergency medicine. This system has added features requested by the physicians which currently are being tested. The practitioner workstation systems are designed to interface with the IAIMS databases and with the HIS.

Icon-Based Interface to the Knowledge Network

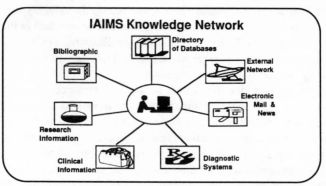

Figure 5.

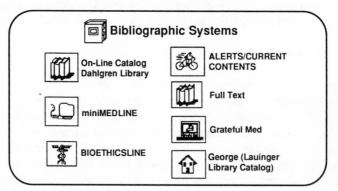

Figure 6.

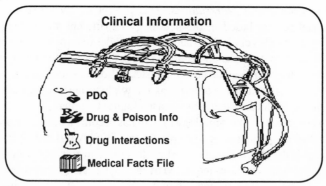

Figure 7.

The Student Workstations/MAClinical Workstations. These workstations are of major importance in the educational program of the schools. In 1981, the School of Medicine began integrating computers in ongoing courses through a variety of partnerships with the Library. Fruition of the student workstation concept occurred in 1988 when the MAClinical and PathMAC projects were launched. A Clinical Informatics Office was established to work jointly with the Library on the MAClinical project.[8] This project places workstations throughout the hospital for student use in preparing history and physicals, and to access the Knowledge Network. Recently, the MAClinical workstations were extended from nine to twenty-four computers. Currently, there are ten workstations for students at the hospital, ten workstations for residents to assist in teaching medical decision-making skills to students, and four at affiliated teaching hospitals for student use during their clinical rotations. More work-stations are planned next year. These stations are equipped with a History and Physical (H&P) report writer program and pertinent HyperCard stacks for student use. Selected sites have ILIAD to experiment with the use of diagnostic systems in clinical teaching. The PathMAC project, originally acquired from Cornell University, has evolved into SuperPATH, a Georgetown-integrated system with digitized images of pathology slides, special lectures, and materials used by faculty. SuperPATH is available at workstations in the BIRC. To facilitate student/faculty communications there is an easy-to-use e-mail system that is available throughout the network to all registered users.

The Researcher Workstation. This project began with two biotechnology workstations designed to provide researchers with integrated DNA sequencing capabilities. It was an experiment to automate the tasks of conducting thousands of sequences in the AIDS research laboratory and for projects in the biochemistry department. The workstations, based in the laboratories, integrate database searching with actual lab work-ups. The concept caught on so well that today over ninety researchers at the cancer center and in other departments use the molecular biology databases and sequence matching software. These systems are available free to all network users—saving access time and expenses associated with dial-up to remote systems.

The Faculty Workstation. This workstation is best illustrated by the IMACS subproject in radiology to develop an IAIMS teaching component of digitized images. We began with fetal anomalies because this is an area seldom seen by students during their training experience. Another example of a faculty workstation is an emerging project to develop a series of clinical teaching materials on diseases that include digitized slides, special notes, and handouts. Once available, these clinical teaching files will help faculty coordinate and update their materials, and students will be able to use the programs for self-study and assessment. Through the IAIMS project and equipment grants from Apple computer, a variety of faculty workstations have been supported. These have emerged as valuable extensions for teaching and patient care. A few are The Mac Embryo in Anatomy, Hyperbilirubinemia Database, Use of Ultrasonography Data Management System in Obstetrics and Gynecology, Interactive Ophthalmic Workstation, Medi-Speak, and Molecular Modeling Software in Pharmacology.

Obviously, for financial reasons, our strategy has been to launch pilot projects and implement a variety of different workstations throughout the Medical Center and then fully implement the most successful projects. To date, from the perspective of high use and return on investment, we have experienced immense success with the student and researcher workstations. We believe the practitioner workstation will accelerate as the HIS completes a Patient Care Information System (PCIS) over the next five years. The faculty workstation projects have been slower to develop because they require an immense financial investment plus staff and faculty time to develop fully. However, the few faculty that have shown initiative are benefiting, because teaching has been made easier for them and more fun for their students.

Integration: BioSYNTHESIS, HIS, and Voice

Academic medical centers need to consider system integration to help their physicians, researchers, and students cope in today's information age and to compete effectively in the current environment. The growing number of information databases and knowledge systems, technological advances and equipment investments, coupled with shrinking budgets, make integration not only a necessity, but the only logical approach to system efficiency. However, the immediate challenge to systems integration for the Georgetown IAIMS is to improve information flow and integrate information within the institution without sacrificing the investment of two existing, sophisticated systems — the LIS and HIS. An important solution has been to use a distributed systems approach that provides major links to institutional computers via the network system, and to achieve system integration in a modular manner by enhancing existing systems. Pivotal to this, is having a well-developed network system, an easy means to navigate through the system, and an interface or integration with the hospital system.

BioSYNTHESIS Software. This software, developed in-house, facilitates access and provides transparent navigation of the varied IAIMS databases. Through BioSYNTHESIS, workstation users already have seamless access to disparate mainframes and minicomputers via the network. The single access menu for users is a key and initial step to system integration.[9]

HIS Components. The HIS components to the systems integration approach have emerged. The ability for users on the HIS system to seamlessly tap the IAIMS databases is available from the hospital workstations. Consistency exists because HIS users also have single menu access mechanisms similar to BioSYNTHESIS and thereby have functional capabilities of both systems readily available at the touch of a single key. A five-year project to greatly enhance the HIS system was undertaken by the hospital in 1991. Plans are to achieve an integrated PCIS that functions as a virtual database of all patients seen at Georgetown. Because of the magnitude of this data, the system will use optical disk technology for storage. The goals of HIS complement those of IAIMS because integration of the medical record, hospital systems, and Knowledge Network resources are being implemented so users can conduct their medical work in a one-step process.

Voice Recognition. This is an experiment of the IAIMS project to collaborate with the hospital's HIS team and radiology on a voice recognition project. We acquired a voice system in breast mammography developed by Kurzweil Applied Intelligence, Inc., and the HIS team undertook the task of developing software to integrate data from the voice system into the HIS central patient record. At this workstation, currently being tested in radiation therapy, the physician can dictate a report and the data is transferred in real-time to the central hospital's system. Another station was placed in emergency medicine for teaching purposes which exposes students to this futuristic technology. Overall, acceptance by the physicians of the voice system has been disappointing. Presently, the machine requires dedication and persistence on the part of the physicians.

Core Support Services and the BIRC

At the Georgetown IAIMS, basic core support services are provided as free as possible to all medical center users. Support is also available to develop educational subprojects within the scope of IAIMS. Access to the databases and network system is free. The Library has emerged as the focal point for medical academic computing. Combined efforts of library personnel (including BIRC and IAIMS) comprise the core support systems team. In addition, there are technical experts in HIS, NBRF, IMACS, and the information systems department of the main campus who often contribute special technical knowledge when needed. The MAClinical project is an example of an IAIMS joint effort in which technical support is provided by the Library and content support is contributed by faculty. Technical support includes developing software applications, acquisitions and maintenance of hardware, and training on use of the workstations. Academic support is coordinated with the Medical Informatics Office in the School of Medicine.[10]

The Teaching Role of the BIRC. Users must be taught how to use computers so they can benefit from the numerous available resources provided by an IAIMS program. A training program is not only desirable but essential. At Georgetown computer training is provided in the BIRC located in the Library. Courses are given regularly and evening classes are often arranged for departments. Information access skills, use of computer-based education programs and basic instruction on the use of personal computers are provided by the BIRC staff. In addition, training is given on database development, personal information management, and the use of factual databases and knowledge systems for medical decision making. Reference librarians play a significant role in teaching the use of databases (see Figure 8).

The BIRC software collection program, begun in 1982, currently includes over 300 titles with multiple copies of popular software. The BIRC staff, who also operate the Center, work with faculty to encourage educational software development. Emerging from joint ventures with the School of Medicine are several pertinent and exciting medical informatics projects. Recent additions are the Electronic Textbook in Human Physiology project funded through a Department of Education grant awarded to the Library and a Microanatomy Digital Slide Library supported with in-house resources.

IAIMS Technology Laboratory Services. As the IAIMS program evolves, a working strategy using subgroup teams for project implementation has

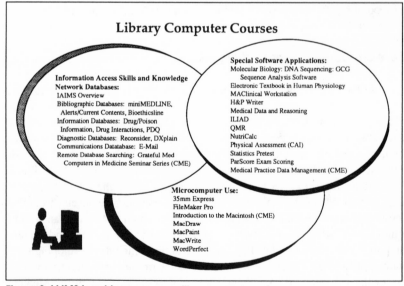

Figure 8. IAIMS teaching programs: library-sponsored

emerged that is proving to be successful. The IAIMS technical staff are assigned to work with medical center faculty who are developing special project components. Planning meetings and brainstorming sessions are held initially; a calendar is established with target deadline dates; tasks are assigned; additional meetings are scheduled as needed; and incremental steps are established for a phased approach to implementation.[11]

Technical Resources

The Georgetown University-wide network system encompasses three major components: IAIMS, the hospital, and the university. The university and IAIMS use an AT&T telecommunications systems as the backbone system with nodes for electronic transmission of data. The IAIMS communications network includes two AT&T ISN nodes which were the first LAN systems to be implemented at Georgetown. The IAIMS network configuration has over 500 end points. The university network has eight ISN nodes, supporting approximately 1,600 asynchronous and synchronous connections. Fiber optic cable connects all of the ISN nodes. The hospital's HIS uses the Sytek system, a broadband network which currently has 1,100 end points. The IAIMS network has thirty-two ports which provide a bridge between the ISN and the HIS Sytek network for a pathway. Users access the network from home, office, or the campus, and they can use the gateway to remote systems.[12,13]

The IAIMS computer network includes eleven host computers: two DEC VAXs, an 8550 and a 6420; a Sun 490; and eight AT&T 3B2 series minicomputers. (These machines will be updated soon.) An Ethernet backbone connects all the machines. TCP/IP provides remote login and file transfer between the VAX machines and the AT&T hosts. DECNET is used on both VAXs, primarily for support of terminal servers. MNET allows MUMPS applications on the VAXs to share files.

The LAN systems at departmental levels focus on AT&T, IBM, and Macintosh microcomputer systems. The Macintosh workstation is emphasized for development of education software and instructional purposes. However, there are ample resources to support IBM PC and AT&T Unix PC users throughout the Medical Center. At the departmental level, several PC networks are integrated into the ISN and Sytek networks. The Novell network system is also available for PC users of the Sytek network. The Novell approach is used in the cancer center. AppleTalk links the Library's Macintosh workstations. To date, the Medical Center has allowed departments to implement diverse LANs which the IAIMS or HIS staff facilitate by linking departments to the Knowledge Network.

The technical team is comprised of nearly twenty technical experts including librarians, information specialists, system/programmer analysts, and electronic technicians who work under the guidance of the IAIMS project director. Approximately ten of the twenty staff are partially or fully supported from the IAIMS grant. The IAIMS Technology Laboratory staff consist of six computer scientists who manage the IAIMS computers, networks, and vast array of peripheral support systems. They are also charged with the development of software for network protocols, system integration, and user interfaces needed for the BioSYNTHESIS prototype. A team of four librarians involved in IAIMS planning and database development work with the project director to explore additional funding sources, develop new databases, and update existing databases. The BIRC staff of eight includes two programmers (supported by IAIMS), computer instructors, programmers, electronics technicians, and a library assistant. There are also two programmers in other departments who were partially supported for over two years by IAIMS, one in HIS and one in radiology.[14]

IAIMS: Results and Observations

During the past ten years, astonishing changes have occurred in the way health professionals at Georgetown access, store, manage, and create information. IAIMS has been a powerful change agent: it has served as a catalyst for integration of various institutional information resources. Tangible outcomes of the IAIMS program have been observed which combine to have a direct impact on the way information is transferred and utilized at Georgetown. IAIMS has served to:

- advance the concept of integration;
- create a high-performance "virtual library";
- accelerate the use of computers to enhance education;
- increase user acceptance of advanced technologies; and
- establish cost factors of providing information resources.

Concept of Integration

Yesterday's information seeker had to rely on a personal arsenal of telephone numbers, access codes, log-in procedures, and searching strategies. Because of IAIMS, today's information seeker is guided through the network and navigates from database to database and system to system in a seamless fashion. A users's effort is spent in using the information, not looking for it. Integration has improved access and utilization of resources, and has served to promote institution-wide sharing of information. In 1983, for example, links to the HIS and the three campus libraries were non-existent. Today, there is greater interest in improving the flow of medical information and providing synergy between clinical, education, and research information.[15]

A High-Performance "Virtual Library"

Nowhere at Georgetown is acceptance of IAIMS in education more apparent than in its high-performance "virtual library." The role of the library and the librarians has shifted dramatically. It plays an essential role in the information infrastructure and it is undeniable that the high-performance computing and communications initiative needs some library participation before it can impact every home, hospital, and school in the nation successfully. Today, the Dahlgren Library serves as a link to information wherever it might reside. As a virtual library it can access information electronically through Internet anywhere in the world. It provides a communications vehicle through e-mail for medical researchers, physicians, and educators. It transfers data through high-speed lines and is working on transmitting images so Georgetown-based research can be shared with other academic medical libraries. High-performance technology is being used to solve complex computer problems.

The high-performance virtual library has a new instructional role—that of teaching the mechanics of information management, information access, and information retrieval which resides with librarians. For physicians-in-training, learning to navigate through information systems to manage knowledge is as essential in the curriculum as course content. The Library is teaching students to perform clinical information tasks such as preparing automated histories and physicals of patient encounters, manipulating diagnostic systems to learn differential diagnosis, looking up drugs, and determining options for treatment modalities.

For the basic sciences, the Library, in its new role, has incorporated high-tech projects to develop software programs to provide students with supplemental learning resources. Projects that have provided visualization of the human system, leading to a better understanding of complex functions of the body, have been given a high priority by the Library. These include the SuperPATH system, that integrates digitized microscopic and gross pathology images with lecture notes, glossaries, and explanatory text; a Microanatomy Digital Slide Library, developed by IAIMS staff, of sixteen laboratory exercises and over 500 images to support a histology course; and the Electronic Textbook in Human Physiology funded by a library grant from the Department of Education and also supported by the BIRC's computer classroom and staff.

In the clinical sciences, the Library emphasized its role as a virtual library by introducing the MAClinical workstations to transform the way students manage and access information. Through these twenty-five workstations, students have gained skills and information query habits they will use in their future medical practice and in their daily clinical activities as physicians-in-training. They have learned to use various resources including miniMEDLINE to solve patient care problems. Another result of the MAClinical project is the ability to track the type of patients seen by third-year medical students on each clinical rotation.[16]

In 1990, the School of Medicine introduced a new course, Medical Data and Reasoning, to prepare second-year students to solve clinical problems. This course would not have been possible without support from IAIMS and the Library. Two diagnostic systems, RECONSIDER (University of California at San Francisco) and DXplain (Massachusetts General Hospital) are accessible to students through the IAIMS Knowledge Network. Individual workstations in the BIRC and the hospital have two expert systems: Quick Medical Reference (QMR), developed at the University of Pittsburgh; and ILIAD, developed at the University of Utah. Both of these systems operate in a textbook mode for reading the knowledge base, a consultation mode for generating advice on patient work-ups, and a simulation mode where students attempt to reach a diagnosis on a simulated patient by ordering tests.[17]

Enhancements to Education

The most visible impact of IAIMS at Georgetown can be seen in the enhancements to health education. Computers acquired through IAIMS funds are used as memory extenders to shift the education focus from memorization to information access. The educational change begins at computer workstations in the Library, the BIRC, and the MAClinical stations in the hospital. A variety of knowledge resources and learning experiences acquired at these workstations has permeated classroom learning in the basic sciences, patient care in the clinical setting, small group instruction during rounds, and self-learning in the library or at home. The information tools available to students for solving assignments or clinical problems are different today then they were prior to IAIMS, and this impacts on the learning process and required skills. To provide these new skills Georgetown has developed a teaching program that embraces the IAIMS-supported Knowledge Network of major information resources and databases. The network's one-step approach of navigating from one system to the next has changed the education paradigm in an evolutionary manner.

Georgetown has added a medical informatics dimension to the four-year curriculum in which students gain the following computer competence:

- basic computer literacy;
- use of educational software to grasp major basic science concepts;
- bibliographic searching of the medical literature to solve clinical problems;
- use of information and diagnostic systems to complete patient care assignments; and
- preparation of automated history and physical reports on patient encounters.

In the School of Medicine, basic computer instruction is part of the required freshman orientation given by the Library, and computers are integrated into eight required courses in Years 1 and 2, and into four major clinical clerkship rotations in Years 3 and 4—medicine, surgery, pediatrics, and neurology. Very little of this existed prior to IAIMS.

Acceptance of Advanced Technologies

An obvious impact of the IAIMS program is the way it has transformed the information behavior of Georgetown's health professionals: faculty, students, and staff. There is a noticeable interest in learning how to incorporate computers in daily activities, how to develop information access skills for life-long learning, and how to search and retrieve medical literature. Despite a stable user clientele, literature searches and use of library materials has experienced phenomenal growth.

Acceptance of advanced technologies is evident by the immense growth and use of the network databases, and increased enrollment in the Library's computer courses. Significant increases have occurred in these areas during the nearly ten years of IAIMS at Georgetown. In 1982–83, there were only two bibliographic databases available to users: the Dahlgren Online Catalog and the miniMEDLINE SYSTEM. By 1992, there were thirteen databases on the Knowledge Network and the choices now extend beyond bibliographic searching to informational, diagnostic, and full-text databases. During this timeframe, users have become comfortable with self-service searching. User searches of the Knowledge Network databases have increased by 35 percent, while librarian-mediated searches have decreased dramatically (69%).

The teaching role of the Library emerged with the proliferation of new databases. In 1982–83, the Library's teaching program offered informal courses and orientation sessions to over 1,000 attendees. By 1991–92, the Library conducted 279 formal sessions of classroom courses, seminars, and orientations, as well as individual tutorials for point-of-use instruction, for over 15,400 users. Of the thirty-two classroom courses offered currently, some are specific to a particular database and discipline; others provide a broader sweep and combine educational software resources and database searching (see Figure 9).

The core support services sponsored by IAIMS and provided by the library staff are heavily subscribed by the Medical Center community. Attendance in the BIRC has jumped significantly from a total of 68,173 persons in 1982–83 to over 157,000 in 1991–92, consultation services on network technology has increased, and database development instruction is growing. Use of the scholar workstations continues to increase considerably, and the number of searches conducted on all the Knowledge Network databases has climbed to record proportions. Figures 9 and 10 attest to the popularity of the IAIMS Knowledge Network databases.

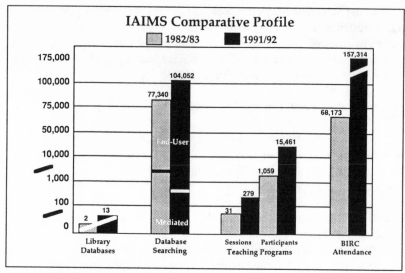

Figure 9. IAIMS impact at Georgetown University: ten years

The sheer number of searches and users accessing the Knowledge Network on a daily basis is an important indicator of usefulness that must be considered. On an average day, over 200 users log into the network. Figure 10 indicates that in 1991 over 148,500 computer logons and over 104,000 searches were conducted by over 2,100 faculty, nurses, researchers, and students. Data on computer instruction and database use shows that over 15,400 yearly users have participated in some aspect of the Library's computer courses. These health professionals, who are extremely busy, devote their precious time to learn and use the network because they receive immense benefits from these IAIMS information resources. Basically, IAIMS offers a fast way to get what they need.

Cost Factors of Providing Information Resources

The provision of information resources in any format carries a high price tag. Choices made must be based on hard data that reflects accurately the information needs of the user.

The IAIMS computer logs provide evidence that the $750,000 grant received from the NLM in 1991 enabled Georgetown to improve the transfer of information to enhance patient care, research, and education at amazingly low costs. In 1991, the Knowledge Network logs show 148,566 computer functions were conducted by users. This raw data shows that each encounter costs approximately $5.05, which is a reasonable cost considering the wealth of infor-

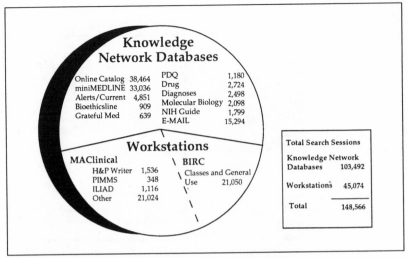

Figure 10. Use of databases and workstations: 1991-1992

mation and benefits received by each user. Incidentally, these figures exclude use and costs of HIS, IMACS, and LIS, nor do they include the institutional support by Georgetown.

Another important fact, is the overall effect of the equipment investment from the grant. The placement of computers in strategic areas throughout the Medical Center and Library has been another cost-effective and efficient way of gaining great benefit from the grant funds. The average cost of each of the fifty workstations (computer, color monitor, and printer) is approximately $5,000. The volume of use of these public workstations is so high (148,566 times in 1991), however, that we calculate an average cost of $1.68 for each encounter.

Detailed use statistics are recorded every time a user accesses a database. The direct costs of providing a database can be examined, matched against use statistics for a specified time period, and analyzed as a measure for return on investment. For example, Georgetown spent $75,810 in FY92 to acquire tapes of nine databases as shown in Figure 11. During the year, a total of 48,412 end-user search sessions of the nine databases were conducted with an average cost of $1.57 for each search session. As expected, the biggest "bargain" in searching comes with the high-use databases. Over 33,000 miniMEDLINE search sessions were conducted at a cost of 38 cents per search. While one of the more complex knowledge systems with lower use cost $9.41 per search.[18]

IAIMS has provided the ability to make decisions from hard data gathered electronically about which databases are essential to the institution's information needs based on use and demand. Today, the Library can track use

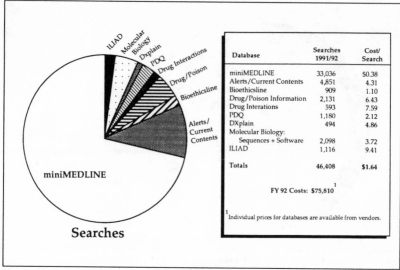

Figure 11. Database costs

statistics and create effective use and cost profiles for each of the resources provided. It has not been possible to have the same depth of detail on use of print resources. With this type of information, the Library can begin to measure value. The need to publicize and instruct users can also be judged by studying activity flow before and after publicity campaigns and courses for large groups. Decisions can be made on whether it is cost effective to continue providing an information resource or whether other options should be explored, such as re-source sharing. With resource sharing, institutions can broaden their user base, distribute and reduce costs, and create a much better return on investment for all involved. Another advantage of having good data on actual costs of an information resource is the ability to prepare realistic budgets and set a fair price for information services.

Conclusion

The emergence of a high-performance virtual library is definitely an outcome of the IAIMS project. Without the initial investment in establishing a medical center network system and developing a digital library with numerous electronic resources, Georgetown would not be ready to play a role in the high-performance information infrastructure that is being developed. The IAIMS libraries are well poised for the next logical step which includes the High-Performance Computing and Communications Act (HPCC) and the National Research and Education Network (NREN). The dream of networking with other institutions on a national system is clearly in the horizon. Already, multi-institutional networking is being implemented among IAIMS institutions. An IAIMS consortium of several universities is providing an initial communications network system for e-mail. It is possible that a major health network will evolve through the emerging NREN and the HPCC recently introduced in Congress.[19] Georgetown is destined to play a role in this network and to find a means for continuing support for the great achievements of IAIMS.

Georgetown's ability to fulfill the IAIMS promise and to carve a role for its library in the future relies heavily on its programs and achievements in recent years. Georgetown needed first to develop the Knowledge Network and instruct a body of users before impact of the program could be analyzed. Credibility has been gained by developing an IAIMS following in the Medical Center, by providing users with free access to commonly useful databases, by giving users training and technical support, and by equipping project participants with start-up systems. Much of the progress achieved in integrating computers in education at Georgetown can be attributed to IAIMS support. System integration for improved information access and information management has been launched successfully through IAIMS. Georgetown has benefited greatly; it has also made a heavy commitment to information technology and this will undoubtedly expand in future years.

As described in this chapter, the project is tremendously ambitious and long term. In reality, much work needs to be accomplished before full implementation can occur. Computers must permeate the entire institution before all the goals of IAIMS can be achieved. New technologies being introduced need to be incorporated. We have a good start, but we know that IAIMS must continue beyond ten years to reach the "ideal" implementation stage.

References

1. N. C. Broering, P. Mistry, and H. Bagdoyan, *Strategic Planning: An Integrated Academic Information Management System (IAIMS) at Georgetown University Medical Center* (Washington, D.C.: Georgetown University, 1986).
2. N. C. Broering, "Beyond the library: IAIMS at Georgetown University," *Bulletin of the Medical Library Association* 74 (July 1986): 249–56.
3. M. S. Blois et al., "RECONSIDER: an experimental diagnostic prompting program," UCSF ACP Computer Workshop, *Medical Information Science* (1983): 7–24.
4. S. H. Grobe, *NEMAS: Nursing Education Model Authoring System* (Philadelphia: J. B. Lippincott, 1984).
5. N. C. Broering, H. E. Bagdoyan, J. Hylton, and J. Strickler, BioSYNTHESIS: Integrating Multiple Databases into a Virtual Database. *Proceedings of the Thirteenth Annual Symposium on Computer Applications in Medical Care*, November 5–8, 1989, Washington: IEEE, 1989, pp. 360–64.

6. N. C. Broering, P. Mistry, and H. Bagdoyan, Biotechnology and Biomedical Knowledge Network: Integrated Academic Information Management System at Georgetown University Medical Center (brochure) (Washington, D.C.: Georgetown University, 1988).

7. S. Potolicchio, J. Hylton, N. C. Broering, and D. O'Doherty, Enhancing Clinical Investigation in Neurology with a Patient Information System. *Proceedings of the Twelfth Annual Symposium on Computer Applications in Medical Care,* November 1988, Washington, D.C., New York: IEEE, 1988, p. 688–92.

8. M. Corn, N. C. Broering, and T. Stair, A demonstration of the MAClinical Workstation. *Proceedings of the Thirteenth Annual Symposium on Computer Applications in Medical Care,* November 5–8, 1989. Washington, D.C., New York: IEEE, pp. 961–63.

9. N. C. Broering et al., A demonstration of BioSYNTHESIS, a system integration tool for multiple databases. *Proceedings of the Fourteenth Annual Symposium on Computer Applications in Medical Care,* November 4–7, 1990. Washington, D.C.. New York: IEEE, pp. 961–64.

10. T. Stair, M. Corn, and N. C. Broering, "First Year's Experience of the MAClinical Computer Workstations Project," *Academic Medical* 65 (January 1990): 20–22.

11. H. E. Bagdoyan, Technical aspects of IAIMS: the Biotechnology and Biomedical Knowledge Network at Georgetown. *Presentation at the 52nd Annual Meeting of the American Society for Information Science,* Washington D.C., October 31, 1989.

12. Bagdoyan, Technical aspects of IAIMS.

13. J. Hylton, Network Architecture of the Knowledge Network at Georgetown. *Presentation at the Twelfth Annual Symposium on Computer Applications in Medical Care,* Washington, D.C., November 1988.

14. N. C. Broering, "Fulfilling the promise: implementing IAIMS at Georgetown University," *Medical Progress through Technology* (1992). In press.

15. N. C. Broering and H. E. Bagdoyan, "The impact of IAIMS at Georgetown: strategies and outcomes," *Bulletin of the Medical Library Association* 80 (July 1992): 263–75.

16. Broering and Bagdoyan, "The impact of IAIMS at Georgetown," 263-75.

17. Corn, A demonstration of the MAClinical Workstation, pp. 961-63.

18. Broering and Bagdoyan, "The impact of IAIMS at Georgetown," 263-75.

19. 102nd U.S. Congress. High Performance Computing Act of 1991 (Public Law 102-194), December, 1991.

CHAPTER 3.
THE UNIFIED MEDICAL LANGUAGE SYSTEM: MOVING BEYOND THE VOCABULARY OF BIBLIOGRAPHIC RETRIEVAL

Betsy L. Humphreys
Deputy Associate Director
Division of Library Operations
National Library of Medicine

Peri L. Schuyler
Head of Medical Subject Headings Section
Division of Library Operations
National Library of Medicine

Abstract

*The National Library of Medicine's (NLM) Medical Subject Headings®
(MeSH) is an extensive biomedical thesaurus used to index, catalog, and retrieve citations to the biomedical literature. It is one of a number of source
vocabularies for the Unified Medical Language System™ (UMLS®), a major
NLM research and development program designed to help users to retrieve
and integrate information from a variety of disparate information sources. The
information sources of interest include bibliographic databases, patient record
systems, factual databanks, and knowledge bases. The UMLS project has produced three new Knowledge Sources: a Metathesaurus® of concepts and terms
from vocabularies and classifications used in different types of biomedical information sources; a Semantic Network of sensible relationships among the
broad semantic types or categories to which all Metathesaurus concepts are
assigned; and an Information Sources Map that describes the scope, content,
and access conditions for publicly available biomedical information sources.
The UMLS Knowledge Sources are intended for use by system developers and
can be accessed by a variety of interface programs to interpret user inquiries,
identify sources of information relevant to these queries, and retrieve the relevant information. A number of specific projects are underway to assess the*

usefulness of the current versions of the UMLS Knowledge Sources and to provide feedback that can guide their future development.

Introduction

For more than thirty years, the National Library of Medicine (NLM) has maintained and improved the Medical Subject Headings® (MeSH), a hierarchical thesaurus used in indexing, cataloging, and retrieving references to biomedical literature. MeSH was perhaps the first thesaurus intended for use both in indexing articles and in cataloging books, and it was also one of the first designed for use as a subject authority for automated indexing, cataloging, and retrieval systems.[1] Among its signal features are: the ability to represent multiple hierarchical contexts for the same term; an extensive system of references from alternate or related terms; explicit identification of the subheadings that are applicable to each term; instructions on how to apply the terms in indexing, cataloging, and online searching; and explicit historical information indicating when each term was introduced and how the concept it represents was indexed prior to that date.

MeSH undergoes substantial annual revision to keep pace with developments in biomedicine and with changes in the usage of terminology in the biomedical literature. Rather than attempting to represent all fields of biomedicine at a uniform level of specificity, MeSH provides a pragmatic reflection of the occurrence of concepts in the literature NLM indexes and catalogs. As the literature related to a particular topic increases, additional terminology related to that topic is added to MeSH. Increasingly, the MeSH development staff also add terminology prospectively, anticipating that it will become important for indexing the biomedical literature. Because it was designed and enhanced for use in automated systems, the structure of MeSH lends itself readily to automated validation of subject heading assignments and automated assistance for subject searching of online files of bibliographic data. MeSH has been translated into at least thirteen languages and is heavily used throughout the world.

While MeSH provides a powerful key to the content of the biomedical literature as represented in MEDLINE® and other NLM bibliographic databases, it is only one of many controlled vocabularies used to describe machine-readable biomedical information. Other vocabularies are used to catalog biomedical books in many university settings, such as the Library of Congress Subject Headings (LCSH), and to index journal articles in systems such as Psychinfo, BIOSIS, and CAS. A great range of terminologies and classifications are used in the non-bibliographic information sources pertinent to healthcare and biomedical research, for example, patient record systems, factual databanks, knowledge bases, and expert systems. The vocabularies used in these sources include the *International Classification of Diseases, ninth edi-*

tion, Clinical Modification (ICD-9-CM), which must be used by practitioners and hospitals in reporting disease statistics or billing for treatments given; the *American Medical Association's Current Procedural Terminology* (CPT) used in the United States to bill for physician-supervised procedures; a number of general or special-purpose vocabularies developed by various professional societies, including the *Systematized Nomenclature of Medicine* (SNOMED) created by the College of American Pathologists; and many locally developed term lists used in specific applications.

The diversity in the biomedical terminology used in different machine-readable information sources and the sheer number of relevant information sources represent formidable obstacles to information access by practitioners, researchers, librarians, and information specialists attempting to serve them. The range of disparate vocabularies and databases also serves as a deterrent to the development of more intelligent search interface programs that could help users retrieve and integrate useful machine-readable information.

In 1986, NLM initiated the Unified Medical Language System®️ (UMLS) project[2] to address the fundamental information access problem caused by the distribution of useful biomedical information among large numbers of disparate machine-readable files. The UMLS project is a long-term research and development effort that involves both multidisciplinary and multisite collaboration.[3] The UMLS approach assumes continuing diversity in the formats and vocabularies of different information sources and in the language employed by different elements of the biomedical community. It is not an attempt to build a single standard biomedical vocabulary. The goal of the UMLS is to build components that can be used in a variety of environments to interpret user questions, to select machine-readable information sources relevant to these questions, to map the user's language to the terms used in relevant information sources, and to retrieve and integrate pertinent information from these sources.

Current Status of the UMLS Project

Following an initial two years devoted to defining the components needed for a fully functioning UMLS and to exploring a variety of approaches to building them, the UMLS project began in 1988 to build three new Knowledge Sources[4]: a Metathesaurus of terms and concepts from a variety of biomedical vocabularies and classifications[5,6] that preserves the meanings and contexts from these existing vocabularies while establishing new relationships among them; a Semantic Network of sensible relationships among the semantic types or broad subject categories to which all concepts in the Metathesaurus are assigned[7,8]; and an Information Sources Map of both human- and machine-readable information about the scope, purpose, access protocols, and so on, of publicly available automated biomedical information sources.[9] In 1990, the first experimental edition of the UMLS Knowledge Sources was issued containing initial versions of the Metathesaurus and Semantic Network. The second experimental edition, released in 1991, includes revised versions of the Metathesaurus and Semantic Network and the first version of the Information Sources Map. The 1991 edition of the Metathesaurus includes about 67,000 concepts and 220,000 terms from seven different vocabularies and classifications; the 1991 Semantic Network contains 131 semantic types; thirty-six allowable relations and 3,481 instantiated relationships between specific pairs of types; the 1991 Information Sources Map describes fifty databases including all of NLM's publicly available information sources.

The plan is to update the UMLS Knowledge Sources annually, increasing their content and modifying their structure based on feedback from those attempting to apply the early versions. To encourage broad experimentation and feedback, the early editions of the UMLS Knowledge Sources are available free of charge under the terms of an experimental agreement that requires the recipients to provide feedback to NLM.[10] As of Spring 1992, more than 200 institutions and individuals worldwide had signed the experimental agreement and received the CD-ROMs on which the UMLS Knowledge Sources files are distributed. The Knowledge Sources are intended primarily for use by system developers and, except for Macintosh-based browsers[11] intended for use by developers, are currently distributed without accompanying utility or application programs.

The UMLS Knowledge Sources and Information Retrieval

The retrieval process is a series of interactions between an information seeker and sources of information. It is a dynamic process in which each exchange of data represents a successive approximation and refinement leading toward an ultimate answer. The success of the process is measured not so much by the quality or quantity of material retrieved but by the extent to which the request for information was understood and acted upon accordingly. This holds whether the interactions are person-to-person, person-to-machine, or machine-to-machine. The classical information retrieval problems of too little/too much or the constant juggling of precision and recall are really manifestations of the basic, but far more complex, issue of concept recognition, understanding, and meaning.

The central hypothesis of the UMLS development is that smart interface programs can make use of the UMLS Knowledge Sources to ensure that the interactions between biomedical information seekers and information sources are successful; that is, to ensure a conceptual connection between the user's query and the information retrieved. The UMLS project is based on the assumption that information relevant to user queries is distributed among many disparate information sources and that, in many cases, a successful outcome will require retrieval and integration from different types of machine-readable databases. The expectation is that a variety of smart interface programs will emerge that will interact with users and employ selected information from the UMLS Knowledge Sources to interpret queries, to identify relevant information sources, and to retrieve and integrate information from these sources. The structure and content of the three UMLS Knowledge Sources have been designed to facilitate both the identification and interpretation of concepts in user queries and the location and retrieval of machine-readable information responsive to these queries.

Representation of Concepts in the Metathesaurus

The focus of the Metathesaurus is on concepts rather than on words, names, or terms. Accordingly, its contents are collected and organized in order to convey the meanings of concepts. At present, the Metathesaurus is established as a "closed world," representing only those concepts or "meanings implicit in the sources from which it is constructed."[12] The information associated with each concept in the Metathesaurus permits a user, a system, or an application to "know" what that concept is, how it is expressed in a variety of sources, what and how other concepts are related to it, and where additional information related to the concept may be found. In the Metathesaurus, meaning is conveyed in many ways—by definitions, by semantic types or categories, by the various words and phrases used to express the concept, by relationships to other concepts, and by information about how the concept has been used. All of these provide for the discrimination necessary to achieve recognition and understanding of discrete concepts.

Concept Definition and Semantic Typing. More than half of the concepts in the 1991 edition of the Metathesaurus contain definitions. This percentage will increase in subsequent editions. To date the definitions have been obtained from the source vocabularies (principally MeSH) or, in a small number of cases, created during Metathesaurus construction to distinguish between two different meanings or concepts that have been assigned to the same name by different source vocabularies. That names are often not sufficient for unambiguous identification of concepts can be illustrated by the term "osteopathy." In MeSH, osteopathy is the discipline of osteopathic medicine; in SNOMED, however, osteopathy is a general expression for bone disease. Therefore, in the Metathesaurus, osteopathy is a name for two different concepts, each with its own definition, and labeled with the appropriate sources, thereby eliminating the ambiguity associated with the name alone. In future editions of the Metathesaurus, individual concepts may have several definitions taken from different sources, such as, MeSH, other source vocabularies, and standard medical dictionaries, each of which will be explicitly labeled as to its origin.

Each Metathesaurus concept is labeled with one or more semantic types or basic semantic categories, for example, Disease or Syndrome, Medical Device, Bacterium. Semantic type assignment is based on the intrinsic properties of the concept and occasionally on its functional properties, as defined by contextual information in the Metathesaurus source vocabularies. Semantic types provide a general indication of the meaning of a concept that enables the accurate matching of concepts from various sources and the discrimination among them regardless of their lexical similarities. Even in the absence of definitions, the semantic types Biomedical Occupation or Discipline and Disease or Syndrome can effectively discriminate between the two meanings of osteopathy. The finite number of semantic types makes them more useful than free-form definitions for automatic identification of important distinctions in concept meaning both in user queries and in machine-readable information sources.

Intraconcept Relationships or Alternative Concept Names. Following on the premise that all words, terms, phrases, or expressions are simply ways to express concepts, the Metathesaurus selects one name as the preferred name of a concept, maps all other terms from the various vocabulary sources that are used to express the concept to this form, and labels the relationship of these terms to the canonical form. For the purposes of retrieval, all terms in the grouping can be treated as identical in meaning. Two classes of intraconcept relationship are distinguished: lexical variation and synonymy.

Lexical variations of the preferred name include spelling, word order, punctuation, and singular-plural variants as well as abbreviations. In the 1991 edition of the Metathesaurus, they are derived directly from the source vocabularies. That is, only those lexical variants actually present in the source vocabularies are included in the Metathesaurus. Future editions of the Metathesaurus are likely to include some machine-generated variants that do not appear in any of the source vocabularies. Interestingly, concepts from the MeSH vocabulary sometimes include commonly misspelled words as lexical variants (e.g., pruritis for pruritus) as well as former spellings (e.g., extroversion for extraversion, kerosene for kerosine). A lexical variant obviously shares key lexical characteristics with the term of which it is a variation. If the preferred name of a Metathesaurus concept is an eponym, then all the variants of this name are also eponyms. The special lexical tags, for example, eponym, trade name, acronym, included in the Metathesaurus identify terms that should not be stemmed or manipulated in natural-language processing.

Synonyms of the preferred name are lexically dissimilar terms that nonetheless carry the same meaning. Synonymy or the equivalence relationship is nearly, but not quite, as tight a relationship as lexical variance, because it is open to a greater degree of interpretation. Since synonyms can be so lexically dissimilar (e.g., Sturge-Weber Syndrome and Encephalotrigeminal Angiomatosis), automated lexical comparison techniques cannot identify all valid synonyms in a given body of terms. Terms identified as synonyms in the Metathesaurus include those designated as entry terms or cross-references in any of the source vocabularies or identified through lexical matching techniques.[13] These "candidate" synonyms were subsequently determined to be equivalent in meaning during review by subject matter experts.[14]

Many entry terms or cross-references in source vocabularies are not actually synonyms. In MeSH, for example, head nurses is an entry term to supervisory nursing, therefore, articles about head nurses will be indexed under the heading Supervisory Nursing and a search in MEDLINE for head nurses will be transformed automatically into a search for supervisory nursing. Despite this close relationship in MeSH, the two terms do not name the same concept. In the Metathesaurus they are not designated as synonyms, but information about their functional relationship in MeSH is retained. In this way, the Metathesaurus supports both precise interpretation of the meaning of concepts and appropriate search strategy development for databases indexed by a particular Metathesaurus source vocabulary. One of the byproducts of the development of the Metathesaurus has been the labeling of the relationship between each MeSH entry term and the MeSH main heading or preferred term to which it points. Within MeSH itself, synonymous entry terms are now distinguished from those that are narrower, broader, or have some other relationship to the main headings to which they are mapped.

The set of the preferred term, its lexical variants, its synonyms, and their lexical variants represents all alternate names of a concept known to the Metathesaurus. Obviously the larger this set of terms becomes the greater the chance that systems using the Metathesaurus can reliably recognize the concept in user queries, correctly translate it into a form suitable for searching a particular indexed database, or search comprehensively for it in a full-text database.

Interconcept Relationships. In addition to specifying relationships among different names for the same concept, the Metathesaurus also represents a variety of relationships between different concepts. These relationships are again derived from information present in the source vocabularies and from lexical matching across source vocabularies, followed by expert review and editing of the results of the matching. In general, different concepts are linked in the Metathesaurus because they share properties or are similar along some dimension. Perhaps the most common interconcept relationships represented in the Metathesaurus are subset-of, superset-of, and instance-of relationships.

The majority of the interconcept relationships obtained from the source vocabularies come from the hierarchical contexts in these vocabularies. All of these hierarchical connections, for example, grandparent, parent, child, sibling, are preserved in the Metathesaurus and identified as to their source. A concept that is present in MeSH, ICD-9-CM, and SNOMED, for example, may appear in several different MeSH hierarchies as well as in one hierarchy in ICD-9-CM and another in SNOMED. As an experiment, the child-parent relationships in some of the MeSH hierarchies have been explicitly labeled to distinguish among those that conform to the pure hierarchical is-a or instance-of relationship and those with other relationships, such as part-of or manifestation-of. The anatomy, disease, and parts of the physiology sections of MeSH have been labeled in this way. If actual experimentation with the Metathesaurus shows this feature to be useful, it will probably be extended. In all the unlabeled portions of the MeSH hierarchies and in the hierarchies obtained from other Metathesaurus source vocabularies, the implicit default relationship between each child term and its parent term is the general narrower-than relationship.

No attempt has been made to integrate the hierarchies derived from different source vocabularies into a single Metathesaurus hierarchy. This would be an impossible task since very different perspectives are represented in the different source vocabularies. The retention of this diversity of perspectives should help the Metathesaurus to be useful in a broad variety of applications. The overall integration of concepts within the Metathesaurus is accomplished via semantic typing and the set of relationships among semantic types represented in the Semantic Network.

Interconcept relationships are also obtained from cross-references or entry terms in the source vocabularies that do not fall into the lexical variant or synonym categories. These relationships are labeled in current Metathesaurus as "broader," "narrower," and "other." The relationship between head nurses and supervisory nursing is an example of an "other" relationship. In future editions of the Metathesaurus, these relationships may be labeled more specifically.

The ability to identify for a given concept a cluster of closely related concepts, to determine the nature of the relationships within the cluster, and to identify the sources from which the relationships are derived offers a significant advantage in retrieving information related to that concept from a variety of sources. Even if a specific concept is not present in the vocabulary used in a particular database, the Metathesaurus can provide a path to a closely related concept that can be a useful retrieval key in that database.

Use Information. Another way to approach the meaning of concepts is to examine how they have been used. The Metathesaurus contains a variety of use information. The current edition of the Metathesaurus contains information about the occurrence of concepts in a small number of information sources, indicating that a particular Metathesaurus concept is present in one or more of these sources. Occurrence information is included for MEDLINE; PDQ® (Physician's Data Query), the National Cancer Institute's file of current information about cancer and cancer treatment[15]; Online Mendelian Inheritance in Man (OMIM), the standard work on genetic disorders produced by Victor McKusick at Johns Hopkins University[16]; DXplain, a diagnostic system produced by Massachusetts General Hospital[17]; and QMR (Quick Medical Reference), a diagnostic system developed at the University of Pittsburgh[18] and distributed by CAMDAT Corporation. For MEDLINE, the number of citations to articles in which the concept was a main point is given. Further information is supplied about the MeSH subheadings that were applied to the concept in these citations, including the frequency with which each subheading was used. For example, the 1991 edition of the Metathesaurus indicates that the subheadings applied most frequently to the concept AIDS in the 1989–1991 segment of MEDLINE were: 2,699 for complications; 1,562 for prevention and control; and 1,331 for transmission.

The Metathesaurus also contains information about concepts that co-occur as main points in articles indexed in MEDLINE. In the Metathesaurus the co-occurrence information can be organized by the semantic types of the co-occurring terms. To use the AIDS example again, the diseases or syndromes and pharmacologic substances that co-occur most frequently with AIDS are shown in Table 1.

TABLE 1. Co-occurrence Information on AIDS	
Disease or Syndrome	*Pharmacologic Substance*
390 Opportunistic Infections	282 Zidovudine
329 HIV Infections	104 Antiviral Agents
254 Pneumonia, Pneumo- cystis carinii	68 Viral Vaccines

The use information in the Metathesaurus has several important potential uses in information retrieval. It is obviously useful in determining in advance whether a particular query is likely to be successful in one of the specific databases for which the specific occurrence, subheading, and co-occurrence data exist in the Metathesaurus; that is, whether a query will retrieve too much, too little, or nothing at all. Beyond this, however, the subheading and co-occurrence information provide insight into important aspects of the concept or issues related to it. This information can be used in interactions with the user to focus or to expand a query.

The particular information sources with occurrence data in the 1991 edition of the Metathesaurus were chosen to illustrate a range of biomedical databases and knowledge sources for which such information would be useful. Occurrence data will be added for other information sources in the future. It is also probable that users of the UMLS Knowledge Sources will add occurrence data for databases of local interest, for example, hospital patient record databases.

Semantic Network

While the Metathesaurus contains information pertinent to a specific concept, the Semantic Network provides information about the broad semantic types that are assigned to the concepts and the semantic relationships that can occur between various types. Its purpose is "to provide consistent categorization of all concepts represented in the Metathesaurus and to provide a set of useful relationships between these concepts."[19] Chapter 4 of this book describes the Semantic Network in detail and discusses its potential uses both in interpreting how the different concepts in a user query relate to each other and in devising search strategies that reflect these relationships.

Information Sources Map

Accurately interpreting concepts and relationships in a user query is not sufficient for successful information retrieval. To complete the loop, a system must "know" where to look for the answer to the question. In the UMLS, information about where to look exists both in the Metathesaurus and the Information Sources Map. As previously described, the Metathesaurus contains information about the occurrence and co-occurrence of its concepts in a limited number of machine-readable information sources of various kinds. Although the Metathesaurus will be expanded to include concept occurrence data for additional information sources in the future, it will never contain this level of information for all machine-readable biomedical information sources. Furthermore, the concept organization of the Metathesaurus is not suitable for storing the full range of data needed to select, connect to, and search automated information sources. For these reasons, the Information Sources Map has been developed to describe various machine-readable information sources that may be relevant to a particular inquiry. For the Information Sources Map, the systematic process that assigned lexical and semantic characteristics to words, terms, and phrases has been extended to databases, databanks, patient record collections, or any other information source. Information is included that describes the specific content of the source at various levels. These include the type of information present (citations, full text, reference text), language, size, updating schedule, and so on. The subject scope of each source is defined by MeSH headings and by the same semantic apparatus derived from the Semantic Network that is used to define concepts in the Metathesaurus. In the case of the Information Sources Map, both individual semantic types and relationships between pairs of semantic types are used to characterize the scope of the databases.

The PDQ database, for example, can be characterized by the MeSH heading "Neoplasms," the subheadings "/diagnosis" and "/therapy," the semantic types "Pathologic Function," "Diagnostic Procedure," and "Therapeutic or Preventive Procedure," and the semantic relationships "Diagnoses" and "Treats." These are expressed as transitive statements, for example:

Therapeutic or Preventive Procedure | treats | Pathologic Function

This approach makes it possible for an intelligent retrieval system to determine which sources may be appropriate to answer a given question. It still does not answer any specific question, however. In the PDQ example, the description of the database does not tell you whether there is any information on the use of a specific procedure to treat a specific neoplasm.

For selected information sources, this last piece of the retrieval picture is included in the Metathesaurus occurrence data. For databases that are represented in both places, the information in the Metathesaurus and the Information Sources Map is complementary. The Metathesaurus indicates that specific concepts are present in a particular database, while the Information Sources Map describes the kind of information present in the database, for example, for PDQ, disease descriptions and clinical protocols, and where and how this information can be obtained. Eventually, the Information Sources Map will contain specific data element definitions and procedural scripts that will permit automated logon to and retrieval from the data sources represented in the map.

Concept recognition and understanding, the determination of appropriate information sources, and the integration of information have been the hallmarks of the UMLS development process. The UMLS project has focused on providing a set of powerful tools that can be used by intelligent interfaces to assist in the retrieval of a variety of data that is expressed in a variety of ways in a variety of disparate information sources.

UMLS Applications

NLM is making use of the UMLS Knowledge Sources in GRATEFUL MED COACH, an expert searcher being developed to assist GRATEFUL MED®[20] users in improving their retrieval from NLM databases. NLM's UMLS collaborators are experimenting with the use of UMLS data in a variety of other interfaces,[21,22,23,24] including several designed to link patient data to relevant information in MEDLINE and other sources such as drug databases and diagnostic systems. Most of these projects involve multidisciplinary teams including computer scientists, medical librarians, linguists, physicians, and other healthcare professionals.

NLM is also experimenting with the use of the UMLS Knowledge Sources in natural-language processing.[25] With information available in the Metathesaurus, the power of a controlled vocabulary can be brought to bear even in searching information sources that do not use a controlled vocabulary or are not indexed at all. Retrieval interfaces can be designed to collect all terms for a concept and search for them in the texts of records in the source. A similar approach can be taken to collect a variety of expressions that characterize the semantic relationships. Incorporating distance measures already used in proximity searching can provide effective retrieval for concepts related in some specified manner.

Although the focus of the UMLS development is on information retrieval, the UMLS Knowledge Sources, and in particular the Metathesaurus, are potentially very useful in database creation as well. There are a number of projects addressing the use of the Metathesaurus in machine-assisted indexing or cataloging of various types of information ranging from bibliographic citations to patient data.

The UMLS Knowledge Sources are powerful tools for the development of more sophisticated and useful information retrieval systems that can provide access to multiple sources of machine-readable information. As such, they have an important role to play in the implementation of Integrated Advanced Information Management Systems (IAIMS) (see Chapter 1). It is probable that the UMLS Knowledge Sources will become increasingly important components of retrieval interfaces employed by medical librarians and by their users.

References

1. S. Gullion, "Classification and Subject Cataloging," in L. D. Darling et al., eds., *Handbook of Medical Library Practice*, 34th ed., Vol.II (Chicago: Medical Library Association, 1983), 268–70.

2. B. L. Humphreys and D.A.B. Lindberg, "Building the Unified Medical Language System," in L. C . Kingsland, III, ed., *Proceedings of the 13th Annual Symposium on Computer Applications in Medical Care* (Washington, D.C.: IEEE Computer Society Press, 1989), 475–80.

3. The current UMLS contractors are: Brigham and Women's Hospital (PI: Robert Greenes, M.D., Ph.D.), Columbia University, (James Cimino, M.D.), Lexical Technology, Inc. (PI: Mark Tuttle), Massachusetts General Hospital (PI: G. Octo Barnett, M.D.), University of Pittsburgh (PI: Randolph Miller, M.D.) with sub-

contractor University of Utah (PI: Homer Warner, M.D., Ph.D.), and Yale School of Medicine (PI: Perry Miller, M.D., Ph.D).

4. D.A.B. Lindberg and B. L. Humphreys, "The UMLS Knowledge Sources: Tools for Building Better User Interfaces," in R. A. Miller, ed., *Proceedings of the 14th Annual Symposium on Computer Applications in Medical Care* (Los Alamitos, CA: Institute of Electrical and Electronics Engineers, 1990), 121–25.

5. M. Tuttle et al., "Implementing Meta-1—The First Version of the UMLS Metathesaurus," in L. C. Kingsland, III, ed., *Proceedings of the 13th Annual Symposium on Computer Applications in Medical Care* (Washington, D.C: IEEE Computer Society Press, 1989), 483–87.

6. M. Tuttle et al., "Using Meta-1—The First Version of the UMLS Metathesaurus," in R. A. Miller, ed., *Proceedings of the 14th Annual Symposium on Computer Applications in Medical Care* (Los Alamitos, CA: Institute of Electrical and Electronics Engineers, 1990), 131–35.

7. A. T. McCray, "The UMLS Semantic Network," in L. C. Kingsland, III, ed., *Proceedings of the 13th Annual Symposium on Computer Applications in Medical Care* (Washington, D.C.: IEEE Computer Society Press, 1989), 503–7.

8. A. T. McCray and W. T. Hole, "The Scope and Structure of the First Version of the UMLS Semantic Network," in R. A. Miller, ed., *Proceedings of the 14th Annual Symposium on Computer Applications in Medical Care* (Los Alamitos, CA: Institute of Electrical and Electronics Engineers, 1990), 126–30.

9. D. R. Masys and B. L. Humphreys, "Structure and Function of the UMLS Information Sources Map," in Salah H. Mandil and Jochen Moehr, eds., *MEDINFO 92: Proceedings of the 7th Conference on Medical Informatics, 1992 Sept. 6–10* (Geneva. Amsterdam: Elsevier, 1992). In press.

10. B. L. Humphreys et al., "Assessing and Enhancing the Value of the UMLS Knowledge Sources," in P. D. Clayton, ed., *Proceedings of the 15th Annual Symposium on Computer Applications in Medical Care* (New York: McGraw Hill, 1992), 78–82.

11. D. Sherertz et al., "A HyperCard® Implementation of Meta-1: The First Version of the UMLS Metathesaurus," in L. C. Kingsland, III, ed., *Proceedings of the 13th Annual Symposium on Computer Applications in Medical Care* (Washington, D.C.: IEEE Computer Society Press, 1989), 1017–18.

12. Tuttle et al., 131–35.

13. D. D. Sherertz et al., "Source Inversion and Matching in the UMLS Metathesaurus," in R. A. Miller, ed. *Proceedings of the 14th Annual Symposium on Computer Applications in Medical Care* (Los Alamitos, CA: Institute of Electrical and Electronics Engineers, 1990), 141–45.

14. D. Sperzel et al., "Editing the UMLS Metathesaurus: Review and Enhancement of a Computer Knowledge Source," in R. A. Miller, ed., *Proceedings of the 14th Annual Symposium on Computer Applications in Medical Care* (Los Alamitos, CA: Institute of Electrical and Electronics Engineers, 1990), 136–40.

15. S. M. Hubbard, J. E. Henney, and C. T. DeVita, Jr., "A computer database for information on cancer treatment," *New England Journal of Medicine* 316 (February 5, 1987): 315–18.

16. Victor A. McKusick, *Mendelian Inheritance in Man: Catalogs of Autosomal Dominant, Autosomal Recessive, and X-Linked Phenotypes*, 10th ed. (Baltimore: Johns Hopkins University Press, 1992).

17. J. A. Hupp, et al., "DXplain—A Computer-Based Diagnostic Knowledge Base," in *MEDINFO 86* (Amsterdam: North Holland, 1986), part 1, 117–21.

18. R. A. Miller et al., "The Internist-1/Quick Medical Reference Project—status report," *Western Journal of Medicine* 145 (1986): 816-22.

19. McCray and Hole, 126–30.

20. R. B. Haynes et al., "Online access to MEDLINE in clinical settings: a study of use and usefulness," *Annals of Internal Medicine* 112 (January 1, 1990): 78–89.

21. C. Cimino and G. O. Barnett, "Standardizing Access to Computer-Based Medical Resources," in: R. A. Miller, ed., *Proceedings of the 14th Annual Symposium on Computer Applications in Medical Care* (Los Alamitos, CA: Institute of Electrical and Electronics Engineers, 1990), 33–37.

22. S. M. Powsner and P. L. Miller, "From Patient Reports to Bibliographic Retrieval: A Meta-1 Front End," in P. D. Clayton, ed., *Proceedings of the 15th Annual Symposium on Computer Applications in Medical Care* (New York: McGraw Hill, 1992), 526-20.

23. J. J. Cimino and R. V. Sideli, "Using the UMLS to bring the library to the bedside," *Medical Decision Making* 11(4 Supp)(October–December 1991): S116-20.

24. W. R. Hersh et al., "Adaption of Meta-1 for SAPHIRE, A General Purpose Information Retrieval System," in R. A. Miller, ed., *Proceedings of the 14th Annual Symposium on Computer Applications in Medical Care* (Los Alamitos, CA: Institute of Electrical and Electronic Engineers, 1990), 156–60.

25. A. T. McCray, "Extending a Natural Language Parser with UMLS Knowledge," in P. D. Clayton, ed, *Proceedings of the 15th Annual Symposium on Computer Applications in Medical Care* (New York: McGraw Hill, 1992), 194–98.

Chapter 4.
Representing Biomedical Knowledge in the UMLS Semantic Network

Alexa T. McCray
Acting Chief, Educational Technology Branch
Lister Hill National Center for Biomedical Communications
National Library of Medicine

Abstract

The Unified Medical Language System™ (UMLS®) Semantic Network is one of three Knowledge Sources currently available as part of the National Library of Medicine's (NLM) UMLS Project. The purpose of the Network is to provide a consistent categorization of all concepts found in the Metathesaurus and to provide useful links between these concepts at the level of the semantic types. The Semantic Network is closely tied to the two other UMLS Knowledge Sources, the Metathesaurus and the Information Sources Map. Taken together, these three Knowledge Sources provide powerful tools for enhancing biomedical information retrieval.

Properties of Semantic Networks

The structured representation of concepts to facilitate computer processing has been of interest to researchers for at least the last three decades.[1,2,3,4] Semantic networks afford an elegant and straightforward method for representing knowledge about a domain of interest. Although existing networks differ in both detail and in underlying assumptions, they all have the following in common. They consist of a collection of basic concept types, which are the nodes in the network and a set of valid relationships, which are the links in the network. The nodes are organized in a conceptual hierarchy, which is often called a type hierarchy. The link between items of greater and lower specificity is generally referred to as the "is-a" link. This link establishes a computer-processable meaning for any given node in the type hierarchy. For example, by traversing the hierarchy from a leaf, or bottom-most node, to the root, or uppermost node, it is possible to assign an interpretion to that leaf node. Figure 1, which represents a portion of the Unified Medical Language System™ (UMLS®) Semantic Network, illustrates the point.

The hierarchical links from Mental Process to Event in Figure 1 show that a mental process is a kind of organism function, which is a physiologic function, which in turn is a biologic function. A biologic function is a (natural) phenomenon or process, which is a type of event. A program can traverse this structure, building up a meaning automatically. This knowledge can then be used to draw inferences of various kinds.[5]

Items in the type hierarchy are grouped either by their inherent properties or by certain attributed characteristics. For example, Figure 2 shows the portion of the UMLS Semantic Network that classifies organisms. The classification shows that a human is a mammal, which is a vertebrate, and so on. This type of grouping is based on the inherent biologic properties of humans.

On the other hand, a population group, which refers to concepts such as Asian Americans, Muslims, and vegetarians, groups individuals according to some particular attributed characteristic, such as their ethnic origin, their religion, and so on. Figure 3 shows that individuals are classified in the UMLS Semantic Network according to a variety of characteristics, including age, profession, or status in a family group.

A concept is placed in the appropriate position in a type hierarchy according to its definition, regardless of whether that definition is based on in-

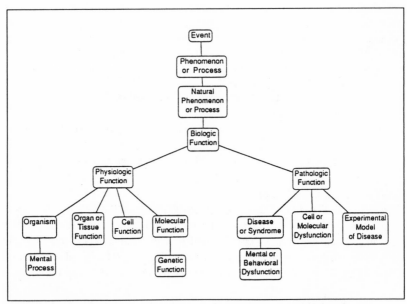

Figure 1. Portion of the "Event" subtree in the UMLS Semantic Network

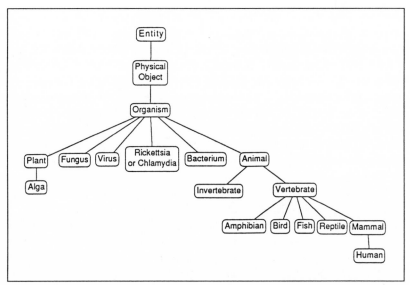

Figure 2. Portion of the "Entity" subtree in the UMLS Semantic Network

herent or attributed features. For example, the type Alga is defined in the UMLS Semantic Network as: "A chiefly aquatic plant that contains chlorophyll, but does not form embryos during development and lacks vascular tis-

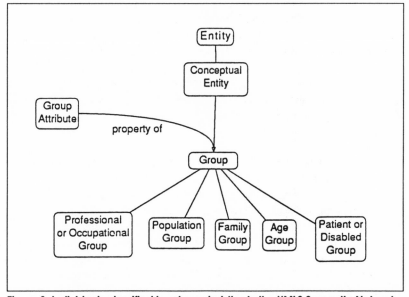

Figure 3. Individuals classified by characteristics in the UMLS Semantic Network

sue." It is clear from its definition that Alga is in its correct position as a child of Plant. All members, or "instances" of the type Alga, such as Chlorella, Laminaria, or Cyanophyta must, of course, also fit the definition. The type Patient or Disabled Group is defined in the network as: "An individual or individuals classified according to a disability, disease, condition, or treatment." Thus, since concepts such as inpatients, amputees, and institutionalized patients fit this definition, they are instances of this semantic type, and are not directly assigned to the semantic type Human, which is reserved for the few concepts, such as homo sapiens, that describe humans in biological terms. Philosophers of language distinguish between the "intension" and the "extension" of a term.[6] The intension is the manner in which a term is described, and the extension is what the term refers to in the real world. The concepts in a semantic network are always arranged according to their intensions.

The is-a link allows nodes in a hierarchy to inherit information from higher-level nodes. This inheritance property ensures efficient storage of information, since information that holds true for higher level nodes need not be repeated for all lower level nodes. The node Biologic Function is linked by "process-of" to Organism in the UMLS Semantic Network. By the inheritance property, the concept types Physiologic Function, Organism Function, Mental Process, and such, are all understood to be linked by this same relationship to Organism and all of its descendants (see Figures 1 and 2). In some cases there will be a conflict between the placement of items in a type hierarchy and the information to be inherited. If this is so, the inheritance of a particular general attribute is said to be blocked for that node. By inheritance, the concept type Mental Process would be said to be a process of Plant. From the point of view of the taxonomy, plants, and mental processes are in their correct positions, but since plants are not sentient beings, it becomes necessary to block this particular inference.

In addition to the hierarchical is-a link, other types of relations between the nodes are included in semantic networks. It is the inclusion of these additional links that distinguishes a network from a simple type hierarchy. Relationships are generally binary; that is, they link two types, asserting a relationship between them (see Figure 4). (All unlabelled links in the diagram are is-a links.)

Several of the types are related by the part-of link; for example, Cell Component is part of Cell, and Cell is part of Tissue. The relationship contains links Fully Formed Anatomical Structure to Body Substance. It is possible to read the relationship with its arguments (the types) as a sort of sentence, or assertion; for example, Fully Formed Anatomical Structure contains Body Substance. The arguments of a binary relation are necessarily ordered. That is, it is true to say that cells are part of tissue, but it is not true to say that tissue is part of cells. However, each relation will have an inverse associated with it. The inverse of part-of is has-part; the inverse of contains is contained-in. Using

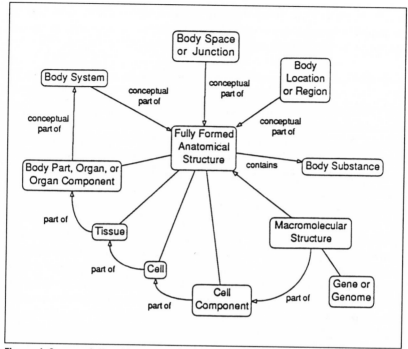

Figure 4. Some relationships in the UMLS Semantic Network

this inverse it is possible to reverse the directionality of the types and to make, for example, the true statement that a tissue has part cell.

Relationships may be stated between types at any level of a hierarchy. All descendants of the types inherit the relationship, but none of its ancestors. For example, in Figure 3, Group Attribute is a property of Group, and of all of its children, for example, Professional or Occupational Group, Population Group, among others. Group Attribute is not, however, a property of Conceptual Entity or Entity.

The relationships that are chosen for a network depend heavily on the particular domain for which the network is being built as well as on its intended use. Most networks would include such general relations as part-of, property-of, affects, causes, precedes, and so on, but usually the domain and application will dictate the full set. By convention, in the UMLS Semantic Network, types are expressed as nouns and relationships are expressed as verbs.

Relationships, just like types, are given precise definitions, and, just like types, they may exist in a hierarchy. For example, in the UMLS Semantic Network, the relation "functionally related to" is defined as "related by the carrying out of some function or activity," and it has several children, for example, interacts-with, produces, affects. Then, since affects subsumes the meanings of three additional functional relationships, complicates, causes, and disrupts, it is the parent of these three.

Evolution and Current Status of the UMLS Semantic Network

The UMLS Semantic Network, like the other UMLS Knowledge Sources, was created in order to facilitate the retrieval of information from biomedical databases. The explicit goal of the Semantic Network is to provide a consistent categorization of the concepts represented in the UMLS Metathesaurus and to provide a set of useful relationships between these concepts. (See Chapter 3 for a description of the Metathesaurus.) The initial versions of the network were developed based on analyses of the vocabularies included in the Metathesaurus and based on experiments using the UMLS test collection of queries and MEDLINE citation records.[7] Analysis of existing structured vocabularies, such as MeSH, yielded a set of high-level categories that resulted in the initial set of semantic types, and work with the UMLS test collection resulted in the initial set of relationships. The queries and citation records were examined to determine the explicit or implicit relationships they contained. For example, a citation record with a disease term such as "Scarlet Fever" qualified by the subheading "etiology," together with the name of a bacterium such as "Streptococcus" illustrates the causes relationship. When enough instances exemplified a particular relationship, then this became a candidate link for inclusion in the network. In this case the link would be stated as follows: "Bacterium" causes "Disease or Syndrome." Concurrently with the work on the Semantic Network, experiments were conducted in making explicit the relationships between MeSH child and parent terms in certain sections of the vocabulary. This led to further candidate relationships for inclusion in the network. After the initial set of semantic types and relationships had been determined, the structure for the first release of the network was finalized. Participation by all UMLS research collaborators resulted in the current form of the network, and continued feedback from users of the UMLS Knowledge Sources will influence its future development.[8]

The 1991 release of the UMLS Semantic Network includes 131 semantic types and thirty-five relationships in addition to is-a. The semantic types are the nodes in the network and the relationships are the links. Each concept in the Metathesaurus is assigned to one or more of the semantic types in the network. Included in the network are semantic types for organisms, anatomical structures, biologic function, chemicals, behaviors and other activities, and concepts and ideas. The scope is quite broad, allowing for the categorization of concepts across a large number of biomedical domains. The level of granularity of the semantic types differs, however. Consider, for example, Figure 2 which shows the type hierarchy for organisms. Subtypes of Vertebrate are included in the network but subtypes of Invertebrate are not. Thus, concepts such as amoeba, protozoa, house flies, and lobsters all receive the same semantic type. The intent of the initial versions of the network has been to establish a set of semantic types that will be useful for a variety of tasks, without introducing undue complexity. In subsequent versions it is quite possible that further distinctions will be made based on the use of the network in actual applications.

Assigning semantic types to Metathesaurus concepts involves algorithmic procedures as well as extensive review by subject matter experts. Wherever possible, default semantic types are assigned to concepts by a program. This is possible because most of the constituent vocabularies in the Metathesaurus are already structured, providing useful semantic information. For example, if a concept appears in the D18 (Cardiovascular Agents) subtree of MeSH, then it is assigned the default semantic type Pharmacologic Substance; or if the concept appears in the C11 (Eye Diseases) subtree, then it is assigned the default type Disease or Syndrome. These default assignments are subsequently reviewed by experts who determine if the correct assignment has been made and whether any types need to be added. For example, the concept cutis laxa, or dermatomegaly, receives the default semantic type Disease or Syndrome since it appears in the C17 (Skin Diseases) section of MeSH. This is correct, but, in addition, the semantic type Congenital Abnormality is assigned by a subject matter expert, since cutis laxa is a congenital skin disorder. For some concepts it is not possible to assign default semantic types reliably on the first pass, either because the concept comes from an unstructured source vocabulary, or because its position in a structured vocabulary does not map easily to a semantic type. If this is the case, the semantic type or types are assigned by subject matter experts. In either case, whether the initial assignment has been done algorithmically, or whether it has been done by a subject matter expert, there is further review to ensure accuracy and consistency.

There are two basic assumptions in the assignment of semantic types. The first is that each concept is assigned to the most specific semantic type available. This means, for example, that a concept such as Learning is assigned to Mental Process, rather than to the more general Organism Function, or the even more general Physiologic Function (see Figure 1). The granularity of the semantic types determines what will be considered to be the most specific type available. For example, the semantic type Organization currently has three children in the network: Healthcare Related Organization, Professional Society, and Self-Help or Relief Organization. There are organizations that fit none of these categories. Rather than proliferate the number of semantic types, concepts which do not fit these subcategories, such as information centers, government agencies, or trade unions, are simply assigned to the more general semantic type Organization.

The second assumption is that semantic types are assigned according to the meaning or meanings that the concept has in its source vocabulary. For example, the concept electrolysis in MeSH refers to the general process of destruction by galvanic electric current, while in SNOMED it refers specifically to the dermatologic procedure of removing hair from the body. Accordingly, the MeSH meaning of electrolysis is considered one concept and is assigned to the semantic type Phenomenon or Process, while the SNOMED meaning is considered a separate concept and is assigned to Therapeutic or Preventive Procedure. The MeSH and SNOMED subtrees make these different meanings clear:

MeSH:

Physical Sciences
  Chemistry
    Chemistry, Physical
      Electrochemistry
        Electrolysis

SNOMED:

Procedure Axis
  Hematopoietic, Oncologic, Immunologic,
  and Dermatologic Procedures
    Dermatologic Procedures
      Electrolysis

A concept may be assigned multiple semantic types within the same vocabulary. This will be the case if the concept appears in different contexts in the vocabulary, and if those contexts signal different semantic types. In MeSH, for example, the concept Factor V appears as a descendant of both Coagulants and Blood Proteins. The first context signals the functional aspect of Factor V, and the semantic type Biologically Active Substance is assigned for this aspect. The second context signals the structural aspect of Factor V, and the semantic type Amino Acid, Peptide, or Protein is assigned to capture this meaning.

The relationships established for the network fall into four major categories which are themselves relationships: physically related to, for example, part-of, contains, location-of; temporally related to, for example, precedes, co-occurs with; functionally related to, for example, causes, carries-out, treats; and conceptually related to, for example, measures, property-of, diagnoses. While the semantic types establish the basic meanings of Metathesaurus concepts, the relationships establish potential links between them.

The relationships link one semantic type to another, but they do not directly link one concept to another. That is, each relationship is stated as a possible link between the high-level semantic types, but for any particular pair of concepts that have been assigned to those semantic types, the relationship may or may not hold. For example, the semantic type Sign is linked to Organism Attribute by the relationship evaluation-of. This expresses the notion that signs are judgments concerning the degree or value of some, generally inherent, property of humans or other organisms. A particular sign or a particular attribute may or may not be linked by this relationship. Thus, signs such as fever, freckles, and bradycardia are evaluations of the organism attributes, body temperature, skin pigmentation, and pulse, respectively. However, fever is not an evaluation of pulse, and bradycardia is not an evaluation of skin pigmentation, and so on. This aspect of the UMLS Semantic Network distinguishes it from many other networks, where the goal is to build a full knowledge base of concepts in a domain.[9,10,11] In those networks every concept in the domain is also a node in the network and is further linked to other concepts by explicit relationships. In the UMLS Semantic Network, the concepts are mapped to the higher level semantic types, and those relationships thought to be useful for information retrieval are established at this higher level.

The following example illustrates an intended use of the network relationships. The clinical query, "What is the efficacy of H-2 blockers to prevent duodenal ulcer recurrence?" might be translated into a MEDLINE query by combining the two main concepts as follows: H-2 blockers (Histamine H-2 Receptor Blockaders) and Duodenal Ulcer.[12] In MEDLINE this search yields a total of 107 citations in the current file and the most recent backfile. This is a rather large number of citations and the search can be refined with the help of the UMLS Knowledge Sources. In the Metathesaurus, Duodenal Ulcer has the semantic type Disease or Syndrome and Histamine H-2 Receptor Blockaders has the type Pharmacologic Substance. Some possible relationships between pharmacologic substances and diseases as stated in the Semantic Network are causes, prevents, complicates, and treats. A user might be provided with this information and asked which relationship was of interest. In this case it would be "prevents." For the MEDLINE search, the program could then suggest that the MeSH subheading "prevention and control" be added to the query. When the search is rerun with this change, seven citation records are retrieved, all of which are highly relevant to the user's initial request.[13] In this case, the network relationships have signalled the possible links between semantic types and the MEDLINE database has provided the actual links between the concepts of interest.

Relationship to the Other UMLS Knowledge Sources

The Semantic Network serves as an authority for the semantic types that are assigned to concepts in the Metathesaurus and that are assigned to databases in the Information Sources Map (ISM). The network defines these types, both with textual descriptions and by means of the information inherent in its hierarchies. It defines the set of relationships that hold between high-level semantic types and, in conjunction with the other Knowledge Sources, makes these available for the purpose of enhancing existing information retrieval methods.

The Metathesaurus includes information about concepts that co-occur as main points in MEDLINE citation records. For example, the concept liver occurs more than 35,000 times in MEDLINE citation records during the time period 1989–1991. It co-occurs with approximately 14,000 chemical and drug concepts, 3,700 diseases, 3,500 anatomical concepts, and 9,000 molecular biology concepts, among others. The diseases with which liver co-occurs are such concepts as liver neoplasms (237 co-occurrences), hepatoma (108), liver cirrhosis (105), toxic hepatitis (73), and others. The grouping of co-occurring concepts by semantic types presents a view that transcends the particular co-occurring concept pairs and allows for investigations of the kinds of relationships that are expressed in the database. For example, liver is an anatomical structure, which is associated in a salient way with diseases. The example just given illustrates the relationship location-of between anatomical structures and diseases.

The UMLS ISM makes use of the semantic types and relationships as one way of characterizing biomedical databases. For example, the ISM record for NLM's Developmental and Reproductive Toxicology Database (DART) is characterized by the semantic types Embryonic Structure, Congenital Abnormality, Organism Attribute, Injury or Poisoning, and Hazardous Substance, among others. In addition, valid links from the Semantic Network such as the following are included in the record: "Hazardous or Poisonous Substance causes Pathologic Function" and "Injury or Poisoning disrupts Physiologic Function." There are detailed textual descriptions included for each database as well, but the inclusion of semantic types and relationships provides a computer-processable description of the databases.

Finally, by linking Metathesaurus terms to semantic types, an overall semantic structure for the concepts represented in the Metathesaurus is provided. Concepts from many different thesauri are included in the Metathesaurus, and often they exist in their own hierarchical structures. The network provides a unifying view of all the concepts in the Metathesaurus, no matter what their origin, thereby allowing both individuals and computer programs to forge a single conceptual path through the disparate vocabularies represented there.

References

1. Quillian is the author generally credited with developing the idea of semantic networks for knowledge representation in computer systems: M. Ross Quillian,

"Semantic Memory," in M. Minsky, ed., *Semantic Information Processing* (Cambridge, MA: M.I.T. Press, 1968), 227–70.

2. William A. Woods, "What's in a Link: Foundations for Semantic Networks," in D. G. Bobrow and A. M. Collins, eds., *Representation and Understanding: Studies in Cognitive Science* (New York: Academic Press, 1975), 35–82.

3. Ronald J. Brachman, "On the Epistemological Status of Semantic Networks," in N. V. Findler, ed., *Associative Networks: Representation and Use of Knowledge by Computers* (New York: Academic Press, 1979), 3–50.

4. John F. Sowa, ed., *Principles of Semantic Networks* (San Mateo, CA: Morgan Kaufman Publishers, Inc., 1991).

5. Cohen and Loiselle derived a fairly large number of inferences for a network with many nodes and a small number of relations: P. R. Cohen and C. L. Loiselle, "Beyond ISA: Structures for Plausible Inference in Semantic Networks," in R. G. Smith and T. M. Mitchell, eds., *Proceedings of AAAI88*, 1988: 415–20.

6. John Lyons, *Semantics, Volume I* (Cambridge, U.K.: Cambridge University Press, 1979), 159–61.

7. P. L. Schuyler, A. T. McCray, and H. M. Schoolman, "A Test Collection for Experimentation in Bibliographic Retrieval," in B. Barber et al., eds. *MEDINFO 89: Proceedings of the Sixth Conference on Medical Informatics* (Amsterdam: North Holland, 1989), 910–12.

8. The work reported by Cimino is one example of the type of feedback that has implications for the further development of the UMLS Knowledge Sources: J. J. Cimino, "Representation of Clinical Laboratory Terminology in the Unified Medical Language System," in P. D. Clayton, ed., *Proceedings of the Fifteenth Annual Symposium on Computer Applications in Medical Care* (New York: McGraw-Hill, 1991), 199–213.

9. K. Dahlgren, J. McDowell, and E. P. Stabler, "Knowledge representation for commonsense reasoning with text," *Computational Linguistics* 15(3) (1989): 149–70.

10. R. Hewitt and B. Hayes-Roth, "Representing and Reasoning about Physical Systems Using Prime Models," in J. F. Sowa, ed., *Principles of Semantic Networks* (San Mateo, CA: Morgan Kaufman Publishers, Inc., 1991), 507–25.

11. D. B. Lenat et al., "Toward programs with common sense," *Communications of the ACM* 33(8)(1990): 30–49.

12. This query was provided by UMLS collaborator Octo Barnett of the Massachusetts General Hospital.

13. For example, two of the titles retrieved after the search was refined are "Long-term treatment for gastric and duodenal ulcer" and "H2-receptor antagonists and duodenal ulcer recurrence: analysis of efficacy and commentary on safety, costs, and patient selection."

CHAPTER 5.
HEALTH SCIENCE LIBRARIES
NETWORKING FOR THE FUTURE:
A CASE STUDY ON RESOURCE SHARING

Trudy A. Gardner
Assistant Dean for Educational Resources
Library of Rush University
Rush–Presbyterian–St. Luke's Medical Center

Abstract

This chapter describes a vision of the library of the future which is beginning to emerge among a users group of a health sciences libraries computer system. The system is the Georgetown University™ Library Information System (LIS), a not-for-profit integrated library system which specializes in health sciences libraries. The chapter examines some of the early cooperative projects of the libraries using the LIS. It also discusses some of the exciting opportunities for network and consortium activity which the users group has been exploring with funding from a planning grant from the National Library of Medicine (NLM).

Introduction

Friends of LIS (FLIS) is a users group consisting of libraries which have purchased the LIS software developed by Georgetown University's Dahlgren Memorial Library. LIS is an integrated online library computer system for health sciences libraries (see Figure 1).

There are twenty-eight LIS user centers of which eight include multisite networked libraries. There are a combined total of forty-three libraries that use the LIS software. Of these twenty-nine are academic, nine are hospital, and four are corporate libraries. Between 1982, the date of the first implementation at two sites in Texas, and 1992, the use of LIS has grown steadily (see Figure 2).

The FLIS users group was formed in 1986 by several early LIS users. FLIS members are comprised of twenty-six of the twenty-nine primary site LIS libraries. Its purpose was to coordinate communications with Georgetown,

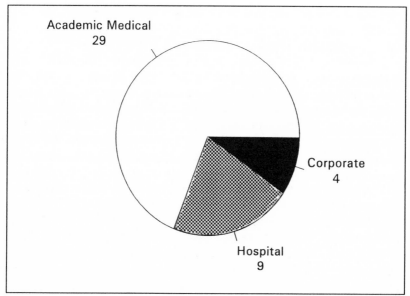

Figure 1. LIS libraries by type

which incidentally is an ex officio FLIS member. The FLIS group accomplished several important activities during its early years: three "white" papers on the need for enhanced LIS documentation, communications, and training; an annual list of hardware at all sites; and a newsletter. On behalf of member

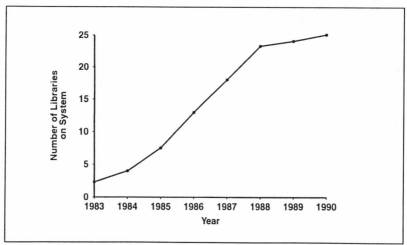

Figure 2. LIS implementation

libraries, FLIS also coordinates and submits enhancement requests ranked by order of priority to Georgetown. Most or all of the above activities are common among user groups (see Figure 3 and Table 1).

In Fall 1988, FLIS members began to prepare a grant proposal for money to plan their future. Members wanted to investigate the organizational structures of other users groups and of other vendors; to look at the successful ones and to plan a structure for themselves. They especially wanted to plan a second generation software that could provide health sciences information for patrons into the twenty-first century. Members wanted to position themselves through planning and cooperation to be able to take advantage of new developments in technology. They felt receipt of a grant would greatly facilitate the process.

Virginia Bowden from the University of Texas at San Antonio and Charles Sargent from the Texas Tech University at Lubbock, two of the earliest LIS users, undertook preparation of the proposal with much help from the membership. FLIS was successful in its application and the National Library of Medicine (NLM) awarded a grant with funding starting June 1, 1990 to the University of Texas Health Sciences Center at San Antonio, with Bowden as principal investigator. As described in the grant application:

> The overall goal of the project is to provide a model of systems planning and development for automated library systems. The project will be a unique effort by a large group of influential libraries to work together to improve existing technology and user services while developing plans for the future. The project has high success potential for replication by other consortia.[1]

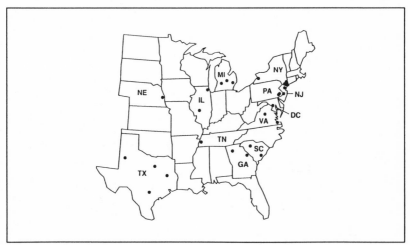

Figure 3. FLIS members

TABLE 1. FLIS Members (26 members/40 sites)#

GEORGIA
Medical College of Georgia
Morehouse School of Medicine

ILLINOIS
Rush-Presbyterian-St. Luke's
Medical Center
Southern Illinois University School
of Medicine*
St. John's Hospital**

MICHIGAN
Catherine McAuley Health Center
Henry Ford Hospital
The Upjohn Company*
Upjohn Business Library**
Upjohn Department Collections**

NEBRASKA
University of Nebraska Medical
Center

NEW JERSEY
University of Medicine & Dentistry of
New Jersey, Newark*
UMDNJ - New Brunswick**
- Stratford**
- Camden**
OrthoPharmaceutical Corporation

NEW YORK
Albert Einstein College of Medicine*
Montefiore Medical Center**
Cornell University Medical College
Memorial Sloan-Kettering
Cancer Center

Payne Whitney Clinic
State University of New York, Buffalo
Winthrop University Hospital

PENNSYLVANIA
Hahnemann University
Thomas Jefferson University

SOUTH CAROLINA
Medical University of South Carolina
University of South Carolina

TENNESSEE
University of Tennessee, Memphis

TEXAS
Texas Tech University*
Texas Tech University, Odessa**
Texas Tech University, El Paso**
Texas Tech Health Sciences
University, Amarillo**
Texas College of Osteopathic
Medicine
University of Texas Health Sciences
Center, San Antonio*
Audie Murphy VA Medical Center**
University of Texas Health
Center, Tyler**

VIRGINIA
Eastern Virginia Medical School
University of Virginia Medical School

WASHINGTON D.C.
George Washington University
Medical Center

\# Three LIS sites are not FLIS members:
   Georgetown University Medical School
   St. John's Medical Center, Tulsa, OK
   Yale University School of Medicine
* FLIS members with multilibrary sites
** Multilibrary sites

The grant has two purposes: to investigate the structures of successful library system vendors and users groups and to develop a vision of a second-generation library system that would serve as a planning document for FLIS member libraries. It is the latter purpose which is of concern in this chapter.

During the first year of the grant AMIGOS, an independent non-profit corporation which serves as the OCLC contractor for libraries in southern states, was commissioned to investigate and report on the structures of five library systems vendors and their users groups. They presented their report to FLIS on June 1, 1991. FLIS members are currently working on ways to follow up on their recommendations.

In November 1990, FLIS members met in Atlanta for a weekend retreat to brainstorm about what a future library system should include. Many ideas were discussed and broad categories were outlined for future investigation by task forces.

Following the June 1991 FLIS meeting, the FLIS executive board with the project grant team named ten task forces to continue the work of the retreat and create a vision of the future system. At this point it is too early to say exactly what the proposal for that system will be. However, there are a number of exciting ideas being considered.

Resource Sharing: Consortia and Networks

One of the most important is that the opportunity exists for FLIS to function as more than an informal cooperative group. Members have already proven they can function effectively as a group, first by coordinating communications with Georgetown and recently by jointly preparing a grant proposal. The NLM grant now enables members to plan the organization's future as a users group and to plan the electronic future of their libraries. More importantly this grant has provided the opportunity to share resources and emphasize access over individual resources.

David Weber, former director of Stanford University Libraries, noticed how cyclical cooperation among libraries has been during the twentieth century. He noted that timing is the key. An idea can only be implemented when the resources or the technology or both are adequate.[2] The FLIS users group is in the ideal position of having both the technology and the resources. Furthermore, because new technologies and networking resources have emerged today in the larger community, future plans are possible.

Libraries are more than warehouses for books and journals; they are vital access points to the world of information. They have a long history and well-established tradition of facilitating access to information by sharing resources and services. This first occurred through informal cooperation, later through consortia, and more recently through networks.[3]

An important method of resource sharing among libraries has been the consortium approach. The consortium was a popular concept in the 1960s and 1970s when resources became increasingly expensive.[4] These consortia were generally local or regional groups of libraries that came together to formalize a governance and organizational structure to share resources and services. A major activity of these consortia was reciprocal interlibrary loan arrangements which encouraged libraries to share resources. Another was centralized cataloging which allowed libraries to consolidate use of staff.

OCLC stands as the most far-reaching cooperative effort by libraries to date. As it grew in popularity it became a gigantic union list of member libraries which attached their holdings to records in its cataloging database. About 11,000 libraries now participate in the network and share over 23 million catalog records.[5] However, even OCLC has lately been threatened somewhat by libraries downloading records into their own databases and not attaching their holdings to the shared OCLC record. Wayne Smith, president and chief executive officer of OCLC says, "While some libraries can cut costs by doing some cataloging chores in-house, that degrades the quality of the OCLC database for everyone."[6]

De Gennaro predicted this course of events in the early 1980s when he said "the interest, energy, and resources that went into network buildup in the 1970s are now going into buying and installing mini- and microcomputer-based local systems . . . ."[7] This has happened even as the need for libraries to share resources through interlibrary loan increased dramatically due to double digit increases in costs of books and journals in the last four years. Costs in other areas—databases and hardware maintenance, to name a few—have also increased while library budgets have stagnated.

These factors must force libraries to reconsider networks and to extend those networks to include sharing newer resources like locally mounted databases, providing interlibrary loan request access to patrons, and cooperative collection development. Harold Billings, library director of the University of Texas Libraries at Austin puts it very cogently. He states, "The growing distance between the quantity of literature produced and the capability of academic libraries to acquire it affirms that the battle for collection comprehensiveness has already been lost. The academic research library model has been changed forever."[8] He continues "There is reason for hope, however. Electronic information is a garden ready to flower, particularly if it will move toward a new distribution, use, and payment paradigm."[9]

The FLIS libraries view the Internet, a supernetwork connecting many local, regional, and national networks, as the highway that can connect our databases and enable us to transmit information including documents. By early 1991 there were 2,501 individual networks (including 757 in foreign countries) that could be reached through NSFNET, the backbone of Internet. Just in the last two years network access has increased by almost 700 percent.[10] Passage recently of the High-Performance Computing and Communications Act of 1991 (PL 102–194) means that the next major network, the National Research and Educational Network (NREN), is close to reality. NREN will provide a high-speed highway for transfer of information and allow rapid transmission of greater volumes of information.[11]

The FLIS Model

For FLIS member libraries, sharing resources though electronic networks will be a viable way to stretch limited budgets and provide enhanced services to their users. FLIS member libraries are uniquely positioned to take advantage of the new technology and strengthen their cooperation because they have a common library system that networks well. Furthermore, as health sciences libraries, members have similar missions and similar environments. Their collections and user needs overlap to a great extent. A closer organizational tie like a consortium, formalizes that commonality and enhances the members' ability to participate in the kind of network envisioned (see Figure 4).

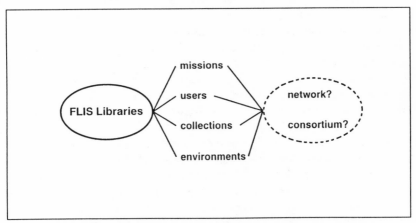

Figure 4. Similarities among FLIS members are the foundation for close ties.

The NLM planning grant allows members to explore a number of options. For example, FLIS libraries may decide it is more cost effective to share access to members' databases instead of every library continuing to mount the same database and incur similar software maintenance and database storage costs. Members may have complimentary files mounted at various institutions such as full MEDLINE or other databases and can provide transparent access to users through the network to the user. A gateway would provide access to databases at several libraries through a menu of choices. The user would only see a menu, for example, of several MEDLINE files with varying dates of coverage or specific areas of emphasis. It might also be desirable to include unique databases in this menu that are mounted at institutions such as the Medis files on CD-ROM at San Antonio or Bioethicsline at Georgetown University. A directory or table of contents database could be included. Numerous possibilities are envisioned; some of which have previously been beyond the capabilities of FLIS libraries (see Figure 5).

The user will not be aware or even care that these files are not based at their home library. To facilitate electronic interlibrary lending, libraries that subscribe to the journals can be indicated in the databases.

There are other library systems that have also mounted databases which "housed anywhere on the network can also appear as locally prompted menu items, allowing users to access what are actually remote databases in the same fashion as those which are locally loaded."[12] This concept is destined to grow as libraries develop approaches for using the new technologies.

Of course, carefully thought-out agreements must be worked out with each institution and with the vendors. Financial and use agreements can be worked out so they are mutually beneficial. Software could be developed to set the maximum traffic on any system at a given time so that such sharing is not only feasible but advantageous to everyone—to FLIS member libraries, to the users at each institution, and to the vendors, who incidentally would generate more revenues based on greater use of their systems.

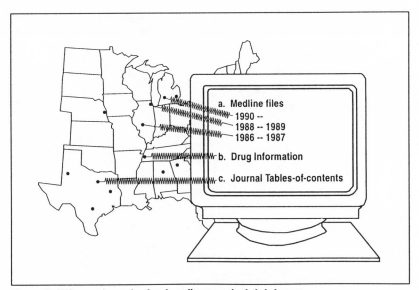

Figure 5. FLIS members sharing locally-mounted databases

A simple quality filtering mechanism to assist the user who feels over-whelmed with excessive information should also be explored. Quality filters have been the subject of research in information science for a long time. However, today there are practical methods that can be implemented. The authors of a paper presented at the June 1991 Medical Library Association Annual Conference recommended quality filter techniques that could be easily made part of database searching. Three of those techniques are:

1. "Quality as defined by methodological rigor of the research design;
2. as defined by some other document attributes, such as research articles or presence of tables;
3. . . . through peer recognition . . . indicated by citation patterns. . . ."[13]

Medical subject headings and other research terms could be made a selection option for users to help identify important articles. For example: Randomized Controlled Trials, Cohort Studies, and Clinical Trials.

Once the user has located materials by searching the databases, the locations of those items may be displayed. For those items not owned by the user's home library, a document delivery module and a gateway to FLIS institutional collections will facilitate transmission of online requests (see Figure 6).

Cooperative collection development is another possibility. Collection development librarians at each institution would also have access to the online catalogs of member libraries. Agreements can be formed for cooperative collection development in certain areas and for dividing up the purchase of unu-

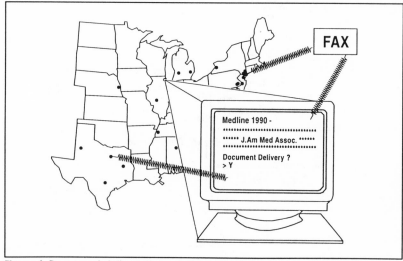

Figure 6. Document delivery through the network

sually expensive or more esoteric works by subject. Used effectively, this could strengthen subject coverage in specific topics. Unlike many cooperative collection development efforts attempted by large academic libraries or by multitype groups, FLIS members all buy materials in similar areas and reaching consensus is easier. Cooperative agreements for FLIS members would probably be less complex than for others.

FLIS members may also want to work with publishers and possibly with a CD-ROM publishing system similar to Meridian Data to produce certain core textbooks in CD-ROM format.[14] It would be imperative that these electronic texts not simply be paper copy transferred whole into electronic format. People need to be able to "read" these books "out of sequence, to browse, to remember what [they have] already seen, to 'write in the margins,' to consult related references without losing [their] place."[15] One public library already is working with Pacific Bell exploring access via modem to electronic books. They currently use commercially produced CD-ROM books but plan to digitize others themselves for dial-up public use (see Figure 7).[16]

Summary

Although FLIS members began cooperative endeavors in order to share information about their common online library system, they now envision ways of extending the LIS system and to use it to share information and resources, to provide additional information access points and even to develop new re-

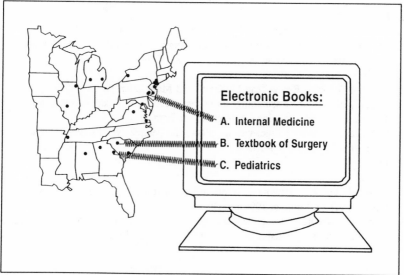

Figure 7. Electronic books on the network

sources. In the future it is hoped that libraries will cease to be evaluated only on the numbers of journals and books in their collections. Libraries must begin to be accountable for the access to information they provide through their interconnections with other sites and "implement policies that favor access over acquisition. . . ."[17]

In a recent presentation a vendor president summed up the current attitude among FLIS libraries today: With today's technology, libraries may be "'stand-alone' but we cannot afford to be 'on our own.'"[18]

References

1. FLIS (LIS Users Group) planning and development grant application to the National Library of Medicine, January 30, 1989.
2. David C. Weber, "A century of cooperative programs among academic libraries," *College & Research Libraries* 37 (May 1976): 205–21.
3. Paul Evan Peters, "Networked information resources and services: Next steps," *Cause/Effect* 14 (Summer 1991): 27–39.
4. Weber, p. 205–21.
5. *OCLC Newsletter* 191, (May/June 1991), passim.
6. "With a flinty management style, president of OCLC trims costs and spurs controversy," *The Chronicle of Higher Education* 38 (October 9, 1991): A29.
7. Richard De Gennaro, "Library automation and networking perspectives on three decades," *Library Journal* 108 (April 1 1983): 629–35.
8. Harold Billings, "The bionic library," *Library Journal* 116 (October 15, 1991): 38–42.
9. Billings, p. 38.
10. Peters, p. 27.
11. Ellen Nagle, "Capital news," *MLA News* No. 241, (January 1992): 7.
12. Rebecca T. Lenzini and Ward Shaw, "Creating a new definition of library cooperation: past, present and future models," *Library Administration and Management* 5 (Winter 1991): 37–40.
13. E. Diane Johnson, Emma Jean McKinin, and Mary Ellen Sievert, "The application of quality filters in searching: some possible methods." Paper presented at the Medical Library Association Conference, San Francisco, June 1991.
14. Reva Basch, "Books online: visions, plans, and perspectives for electronic text," *Online* 15 (July 1991): 13–23.
15. Basch, p. 19.
16. Basch, p. 22.
17. Robert Heterick, "Networked information: what can we expect and when?" *Cause/Effect* 13 (Summer 1990): 9–12.
18. Stephen E. Arnold, "Storage technology: A review of options and their implications for electronic publishing," *Online* 15 (July 1991): 39–51.

Chapter 6.
LIS Net: A Next-Generation Health Sciences Library System Based on Client-Server Architecture

Robert Larson
Coordinator, Library Computer Services
Georgetown University Medical Center

Abstract

It is necessary for hospitals and medical centers to automate their health science libraries with systems that can integrate easily to their clinical information systems. Stand-alone systems, incapable of networking, cannot meet the needs of a highly networked hospital. Physicians and nurses need remote access to medical literature from the clinical setting, home, or office. Cost factors have been a deterrent to small libraries in hospitals that function on low budgets. LIS Net has emerged from the original Georgetown University™ Library Information System (LIS) as a possible solution. This newest and most innovative addition to the LIS system provides not only a new low-cost/high-performance hardware platform, but also enhanced networking capabilities that allow multiple CPUs to share data and distribute workload. Coupled with the new platform is new workstation software which provides a graphical user interface into the familiar Online Catalog, miniMEDLINE SYSTEM™, and ALERTS™/Current Contents® systems. It implements the server of a fully integrated system on new hardware platforms that allows expansion of databases on low-cost workstations.

LIS Net, the next-generation LIS software and hardware, is being implemented as a client-server model utilizing loosely coupled microcomputers as database servers with PCs and Macintosh microcomputers as client workstations. Network access is heavily integrated into LIS design to provide remote user access, to facilitate resource sharing among libraries, to provide timely updates of software, and to directly link library journal subscription and book agents. It also has an e-mail and electronic news component for library-related messages. This modular approach to hardware/software/network design can allow hospitals to automate their medical libraries at one-tenth the current hardware costs by running servers to support many gigabytes of data. Leading-edge technologies used in LIS functions including networking features, graphical interfaces, and new system architecture are described in this chapter.

Background

The Georgetown University™ Library Information System (LIS) is an integrated library system[1,2] designed and implemented to meet the needs of health sciences libraries. It was developed at the Dahlgren Memorial Library, Georgetown University to meet operational and user needs. LIS' functional components consist of nine user-friendly modules: catalog, circulation, acquisitions, serials, bibliographic management (including the miniMEDLINE SYSTEM™), reserves, electronic news/e-mail, networking/document delivery, and word processing for report generating and Help screens. The LIS has computer networking capability which brings the library directly to users through personal or institutional computers at remote sites. LIS is operating at over forty academic medical center, pharmaceutical, and hospital libraries through cooperative license maintenance agreements with Georgetown.

An Update of LIS Modules

LIS has been previously reported in the literature,[3,4,5] but the modules have undergone major enhancements to warrant an update of its current functions. The system is currently operating under version 4.4 and new components have been added since LIS was last reported. One of the most significant additions to LIS is the multiple library version; it has a unique approach for a main library to add branches or other institutional libraries to its central computer system. Another attractive feature is its capability to easily integrate medically related databases such as miniMEDLINE, BIOETHICSLINE™, ALERTS™/Current Contents®, drug information systems, and document delivery to meet user needs.

Overall, the features which LIS users favor have been maintained in the new version; it is menu driven with one entry point. A conscious effort to use clean screen displays throughout the system continues, even as new components are added.

The Online Public Catalog (OPAC)

The catalog contains records of the Library's holdings, including books, journals, and audiovisuals. It provides users with a dictionary as well as a divided catalog for accessing holding information. The search points—which include keyword (Boolean AND), Author, Title, and Subject (Boolean OR)—have been enhanced extensively. There are three levels of record display, but now users have more search capabilities. The first two are an abbreviated display and a full display that replicates the card catalog and contains the call number as well as the circulation status and location of the item. The third is a detailed MARC record display used primarily by the cataloger for maintenance of the master bibliographic file. MARC records enter the system via magtape, online transfer from OCLC, or direct keyboard input. The record is then modified as needed and stored in LIS. A CD-ROM backup catalog has been added to replace or supplement the old computer output microfilm version.

Circulation

All standard circulation functions such as check-in, check-out, renewals, holds, overdues, fine notices, patron notices, inquiry, and reports have been expanded. The major files are comprised of patron and item files (books, journals, or audiovisuals) with barcode cross-reference. Management reports on patron use and extensive statistical gathering are included. An IBM PC-based backup circulation system has been added to collect circulation transaction data when the main system is down and to upload and file these transactions when the main system is again operational.

Acquisitions

This component is totally integrated with LIS. It interfaces with the circulation system for the item file and with the OPAC so patrons are immediately aware of on-order or in-process items. It also provides a single point for pre-order searching by staff. The acquisitions module contains files for regular and standing orders, vendors, and fiscal transactions. It produces order, claim, cancel, and return forms and provides fiscal reports and statistical data.

Serials

The serials component is MARC based. It allows the Library to maintain journal bibliographic records that follow national standards. There is also a capability to output holdings data for the National Library of Medicine (NLM) DOCLINE database. A major advantage of a fully integrated serials control system is that, the instant new issues are received and checked in, the information is immediately accessible to the public in the online catalog. Other special features of the serials component include subject searching, claiming, binding control, routing, and capabilities to load subscription data from vendor invoice tapes.

Networking/Document Delivery

The networking feature allows users to dial-up to the system from remote sties. As an outgrowth of a small interlibrary loan request function developed for local use, a full-service document delivery service, which allows both individual users and other libraries to request loans or photocopies has been developed and is being tested. Documents can be transmitted via fax-mail directly to users.

Reserves

This module is more appropriate to teaching hospitals and medical school libraries. It includes special capabilities for handling items, such as reprints, which are not included in the master bibliographic file. Patrons may search reserves through the main catalog menu by course name, course number, instructor, author, or title. Reserve lending is handled through the circulation module.

LIS Mail and Electronic News

LIS Mail, the e-mail component of LIS, offers the traditional message-sending capabilities between library users. Additionally, a conferencing mode allows a group of users to maintain a continuing dialog on a topic of interest. LIS modules use LIS Mail to communicate library information to users. The circulation module prints electronic overdue notices to users, the document delivery system can notify a user when an interlibrary loan book is ready for pick up, and librarians can do mailings to selected groups of library users. The Library can input in Electronic News any important messages for users. For example Clinical Alerts provided by NIH/NLM are entered in the system as soon as they are received from NLM.

Word Processing

This feature is useful for preparing major documents where more than one individual participates in writing the manuscript. LIS Help screens are developed and maintained in the word processor. It allows individual libraries to edit the screens, if desired.

Value-Added Bibliographic Databases

LIS Net is ideal for libraries that want to implement in-house bibliographic and information databases in their library services. Databases, such as miniMED-LINE, ALERTS/Current Contents, and BIOETHICSLINE, offer the opportunity to give users access to additional services from the main LIS menu.

miniMEDLINE SYSTEM

The miniMEDLINE SYSTEM provides access to a subset of the NLM MEDLINE file Georgetown subscribes to the NLM MEDLINE tapes and converts the records to the miniMEDLINE format which is updated monthly. It is a collection-oriented, in-house system designed for users seeking basic information in the core journal literature for education and patient care needs. Once a small file, today the database contains over 1,000 journal titles, including abstracts covering the current five years.[6]

The miniMEDLINE SYSTEM is clearly the "front runner" in popularity with users. Experiencing almost overnight success in the first two years (1982–84), miniMEDLINE clocked almost 4,000 hours and over 28,000 searches. Use data shows that in the most recent two-year period (1989–1990), user searches have increased to over 39,000.

Because miniMEDLINE is maintained in the Library's dedicated computers, it is available free to registered Georgetown Library borrowers, twenty-four hours a day for users with home computers and all hours the Library is open through in-house terminals. There are also access sites throughout the Medical Center—in each of the schools (nursing, medical, and the Graduate School in Basic Sciences) and in the university hospital. Expanded remote access capabilities have been implemented through the Integrated Advanced Information Management System (IAIMS) network.

ALERTS/Current Contents Search System

The ALERTS/Current Contents Search System is based on a subset of the Institute for Scientific Information's (ISI) Current Contents database, which contains an index of the latest articles in scientific subjects published in journals. Abstracts of the article references were recently added using the new client-server hardware platform of LIS Net. The ALERTS/Current Contents interface software uses bibliographic retrieval routines similar to those of miniMEDLINE. Search access is by author, title work, or journal. It displays single or combined sets with Boolean operators and automatically prints lists of references selected by the user. It has additional features such as the ability to store a search strategy for use at a later date, search by institution or corporate name, and focus on a journal issues contents. Current Contents has five sections: Biology and Environmental Sciences, Chemical and Earth Sciences, Clinical Practice, Life Sciences, and Technology and Applied Science. It has gained popularity with basic and clinical science researchers of the Medical Center.[7]

BIOETHICSLINE

BIOETHICSLINE is the latest bibliographic system added to LIS Net. It is comprised from the NLM BIOETHICSLINE but has the common searching approach of miniMEDLINE and ALERTS/Current Contents. It is used heavily by medical students who are required to write papers in bioethics.[8]

Multiple Library System (MLS)

Multiple Library System (MLS) is a network version which enables libraries to share a computer system with another library. Affiliated libraries elected for inclusion in the network share a master bibliographic file, while maintaining their own patron and item files. With this approach users can easily search the catalog of each affiliated or branch library and also the union catalog of the libraries participating in the network. This allows users to search catalogs residing on a networked computer.

LIS Net Architecture

LIS Net, the newest and most innovative addition to the LIS system, provides not only a new low-cost/high-performance hardware platform for the LIS system but also provides enhanced networking capabilities that allow multiple CPUs to share data and distribute workload. Coupled with the new platform is new workstation software which provides a graphical user interface into the familiar online catalog, miniMEDLINE, BIOETHICSLINE, and ALERTS/Current Contents systems. Taken together the hardware and software innovations transform the LIS model from a centralized computer accessed through VT-100 compatible terminals to a client-server model accessed via personal workstations. The NET part of LIS Net refers not only to the networked nature of the hardware platform and workstation access, but also to networking capabilities beyond the confines of the library and its parent institution.

LIS continues to be ANSI MUMPS based, but utilizes recent advances in networked MUMPS. The Open MUMPS Interconnect (OMI), standards allow for interfacing multivendor implementations of MUMPS and even access to library data by non-MUMPS applications. LIS is thus able to utilize ten years of solid MUMPS and application experience and still take advantage of the latest innovation in hardware and networking.[9]

Modularity and low cost are the key to the LIS Net hardware platform. The module is based on Intel microcomputers linked together with a high-speed local area network (LAN).[10] Libraries can add CPU modules as the library collection grows, as new LIS functions are added, or as the user base expands. The functional modularity allows one module to be disabled while the rest of the system operates normally.

LIS Net hardware is inexpensive and easy to upgrade. System administration is minimized compared to a mini- or mainframe computer by the use of simple hardware and operating system. Expandability ranges from a single server for a small hospital library to dozens of servers and client workstations suitable for the large biomedical institution.

LIS Net supports three types of user interface:

1. At the simplest level is VT-100 serial access which allows backward compatibility for existing LIS customers.
2. There is also a PC workstation running MUMPS. This level allows significant off-loading of CPU resources from the database server to the PC.
3. At the highest level of access, LIS Net provides for PC and Macintosh workstations. At this level there is the off-loading of level 2 but also a graphic interface for users. (Access is written with object-oriented tools which provide easy update and customization.)

Workstations will allow libraries to customize the library environment with non LIS applications and therefore take advantage of low-cost and powerful DOS and Macintosh applications. For example, LIS reports can be downloaded to a spreadsheet for further manipulation. Since most institutions already have an installed base of PCs and/or Macs, the workstation access allows them to utilize their investment, lowering library system costs and providing users with familiar access tools (see Figure 1).

Future LIS Net Features

In the future, LIS libraries will be able to report problems and get software updates online. An expert system will run on LIS Net platforms and relay po-

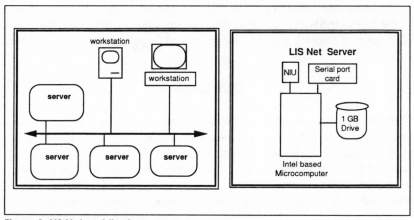

Figure 1. LIS Net architecture

tential problems back to the LIS maintenance team at Georgetown via the network. Interlibrary loan information gathered by the document delivery system will be filed electronically to other institutions. Resource sharing with non-LIS sites can be accommodated through the use of special workstation interface programs which can be customized by the library itself. Bidirectional links with journal vendors can be accomplished through LIS Net. Claims are filed electronically by the journal module and verification returned in LIS Mail.

LIS and IAIMS: BioSYNTHESIS

Having LIS in place has been advantageous to the Georgetown IAIMS project. LIS serves as a hub for IAIMS activities and has inspired development of projects that have led to recent grant awards. The two systems (LIS and IAIMS) have become almost synonymous. The special IAIMS databases harmoniously link to LIS databases. Together they have evolved into a useful decision-support system for Medical Center students, researchers, and practitioners seeking information for improved patient care.

BioSYNTHESIS is an intelligent retrieval system that provides the system bridge. It provides a single menu to multiple databases so users can easily navigate through the system to find the information they need. It is an interface system that can retrieve information based on disparate computer systems. It links heterogeneous computers such as DEC, AT&T, and Sun computers where the various in-house databases reside.

LIS at Other Libraries

What began as a system designed to meet the needs of the Dahlgren Library at Georgetown has been shared with other institutions since 1982. Today, nearly forty libraries use LIS or a portion of it such as miniMEDLINE. The majority of the LIS-user libraries are academic medical libraries. However, there are eight hospital libraries and two pharmaceutical firms that also use the system (see Table 1).

Conclusion

Considerable time and effort is devoted to sharing knowledge, so others can benefit from Georgetown's experience and to monitoring and modifying the system to achieve the greatest possible excellence. The recent LIS Net features resulting from Georgetown's research and development efforts can provide a useful, low-cost solution to hospitals wanting to automate their libraries using an integrated approach with the clinical information system. LIS Net offers a natural bridge capability that brings the medical literature directly to health practitioners wherever they are—clinical setting, home, lab, office, or the library.

TABLE 1. Health Sciences Libraries Using LIS

Albert Einstein College of Medicine; Montefiore Medical Center
Catherine McAuley Health Center
Cornell University Medical College; Memorial Sloan-Kettering Cancer Center; Payne Whitney Clinic
Eastern Virginia Medical School
George Washington University Medical Center
Georgetown University Medical Center
Hahnemann University
Henry Ford Hospital
Medical College of Georgia
Medical University of South Carolina
Morehouse School of Medicine
OrthoPharmaceutical Corporation; Multi-Media Center; R.W. Johnson Pharmaceutical Research Institute
Rush-Presbyterian–St. Luke's Medical Center; Learning
Resource Center; Rush University
St. John's Medical Center, Inc.
State University of New York, Buffalo
Southern Illinois University
Texas College of Osteopathic Medicine
Thomas Jefferson University
Texas Tech Health Sciences Center; Texas Tech University RAHC
University of Nebraska Medical Center
University of South Carolina
University of Medicine & Dentistry of New Jersey
University of Tennessee, Memphis
University of Texas Health Sciences Center at San Antonio; Audie Murphy VA Medical Center; University of Texas Heath Center at Tyler
University of Virginia
The Upjohn Company
Winthrop University Hospital
Yale University

References

1. Charles M. Goldstein and Richard S. Dick, "The integrated library system, version 1.0," *NLM News* 35 (September 1980): 1–3.
2. Charles M. Goldstein, "Integrated library systems," *Bulletin of the Medical Library Association* 71 (July 1983): 308–11.
3. Naomi C. Broering, "The Georgetown University Library Information System (LIS): A minicomputer-based integrated library system," *Bulletin of the Medical Library Association* 71 (July 1983): 317–23.
4. Naomi C. Broering, "An affordable microcomputer library information system developed by Georgetown University," *Microcomputer for Information Management* 1 (December 1984): 269–83.

5. Naomi C. Broering, "Emergence of an electronic library: A case study of the Georgetown University Library Information System," *Science and Technology Libraries* 5 (April 1985): 1-10.

6. Naomi C. Broering, "The miniMEDLINE SYSTEM™: A library-based end-user search system," *Bulletin of the Medical Library Association* 73 (April 1985): 138–45.

7. Naomi C. Broering and B. Cannard, "Building bridges: LIS-IAIMS-BioSYN-THESIS," *Special Libraries* 79 (Fall 1988): 302–13.

8. BIOETHICSLINE is the NLM BIOETHICS®.

9. OMI Document. MDCH X11/SC7/91-1. MUMPS Users Group.

10. Peter D. Beaman and John J. Althous, "An efficient MUMPS distributed database using a high-level LAN Interface," *MUG Quarterly* 19 (Fall 1989): 31.

CHAPTER 7.
ESSENTIAL FUNCTIONS IN AN ELECTRONIC
DOCUMENT DELIVERY SYSTEM

George R. Thoma
Chief, Communications Engineering Branch
Lister Hill National Center for Biomedical Communications
National Library of Medicine

Frank L. Walker
Communications Engineering Branch
Lister Hill National Center for Biomedical Communications
National Library of Medicine

Abstract

Online bibliographic databases have been available for the search and retrieval of citations to the literature in medicine and other fields for thirty years. Yet to this day it is often a substantial effort to follow up an electronic citation search with the physical delivery of the actual documents (or document surrogates). This manual process usually entails the physical retrieval of the paper documents from the shelves, then mailing the documents, or photocopying them and mailing the photocopies, all which are labor intensive and cause delays in the user receiving the requested documents.

Active research is proceeding in automated document delivery techniques, such as, methods for linking a conventional online search of a bibliographic database to the automated access and retrieval of the document itself. This chapter describes a prototype system that serves as a proof-of-concept demonstration of the necessary functions. The system design permits a user located virtually anywhere to search a medical bibliographic database, receive citations, and for the citations of interest, to request the corresponding documents from a central electronic store. The system retrieves the documents automatically and transmits them via facsimile to the user. Though the implementation described is oriented toward biomedicine, involving as it does MEDLINE® and GRATEFUL MED®, the basic model has general applicability.

Introduction

To introduce automation in document delivery, the Lister Hill National Center for Biomedical Communications, an R&D division of the National Library of Medicine (NLM), is conducting research into the hardware, software, and functionality of systems that deliver document images with little human intervention.

Though often used synonymously, automated document delivery in the present context means more than electronic document transmission. Examples of electronic document transmission are conventional fax and systems such as Ariel[1] that employ Internet in place of the telephone system to transmit images. In our definition, the starting point for automated document delivery is an on-line search of the literature initiated by a user, for example, the search of MEDLINE® using computer-based front-end software such as GRATEFUL MED®. (MEDLINE is a database of citations to more than 3,500 biomedical journals, whose articles are indexed by NLM. GRATEFUL MED is a widely used personal computer software interface to the NLM databases.) This search is followed by the delivery of citations to the user who reviews them and makes a selection. At this point a request for the document is sent to a system that holds digital images of a collection of documents. The request activates an automated retrieval of the relevant document image files that are reformatted for transmission, and then electronically transmitted to the user. This transmission may be over telephone channels (e.g., Group 3 fax) or some network, either a local area network (LAN) such as Ethernet or a wide area network (WAN) such as Internet.

Lister Hill Center projects underway include both direct and indirect document delivery. Direct document delivery implies that the end-user, a health professional for example, does a search at a workstation, requests a document from among the citations that result from the search, and gets a digital image of the document directly from a central electronic store. Indirect document delivery, on the other hand, involves the request (automatically) going to one or more libraries participating in a network of cooperating libraries one of which fills the request. The model for this latter approach would use the DOCLINE system of the NLM. DOCLINE, residing in NLM's mainframe computer, is NLM's automated interlibrary loan request and referral system through which more than 2,000 participating libraries request documents from member libraries. DOCLINE routes each request to a library whose holdings show that it has the requested document. If the library cannot fill the request, DOCLINE routes the request automatically to another library. To the end-user, the main difference between direct and indirect document delivery is the longer time required to get a document in the latter approach.

While the indirect system has advantages for a family of cooperating libraries such as the National Network of Libraries of Medicine (NN/LM) administered by the NLM,[2] the direct approach would be more suitable for a library serving a well-defined local user community. Since this is a more general model, the discussion in this chapter is confined to the direct approach, though both approaches have many subsystems and functions in common. The prototype of a direct document delivery system developed at the Lister Hill Center is the Electronic Document Delivery System (EDDS).

Overall System and Operations Description

The prototype EDDS exploits image technologies such as document scanning, digital optical disk storage, LANs, image compression, fax, and high-resolution image display devices. EDDS relies on three major components: the Document Request Workstation (DRW) at the user site, the Document Retrieval and Transmission System (DRTS) that includes an electronic store of document images at a central location, and the NLM mainframe that contains MEDLINE and other bibliographic databases.

The sequence of operations is as follows. First, the user, at any location accessible over the public telephone system, searches MEDLINE via GRATEFUL MED. The NLM mainframe delivers a list of relevant citations that GRATEFUL MED downloads from MEDLINE to the hard disk in the user's computer. Then, through the DRW software, the user may display all received citations and choose from among them the citations for which the user wants the actual article. The user specifies the form in which the article is to be delivered: by fax, mail, or by personal pickup at the central location. The DRW then calls the DRTS, which checks its database of documents that electronically reside on optical or magnetic disks. If the requested documents are in electronic form, they are retrieved from storage, formatted in CCITT Group 3 format, and automatically transmitted to the user's fax machine, or printed out at the DRTS for mail or pickup. If the requested documents are not in electronic form, a request is printed out for an operator to retrieve the paper documents from the collection. These documents are scanned, then printed or faxed, and stored electronically to permit automated retrieval to fill subsequent requests.

Description of the Subsystems Comprising EDDS

The three main components of EDDS appear in Figure 1: the NLM mainframe running MEDLINE, the DRW available to the user, and the DRTS. The NLM mainframe is an IBM system that provides access to more than twenty databases, including MEDLINE. The hardware required for the other two components, entirely off-the-shelf and therefore affordable, is described below.

The DRW hardware consists of a personal computer running MS-DOS, a Hayes-compatible modem, and a facsimile machine. The modem is used to

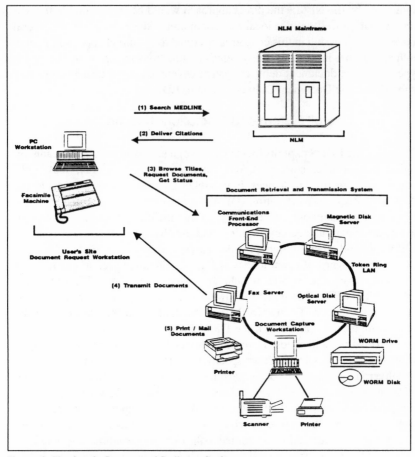

Figure 1. Electronic Document Delivery System

call the NLM mainframe to search MEDLINE, and the DRTS to request documents. The fax machine, a standard Group 3 device, receives and prints documents transmitted by the DRTS.

The DRTS is a complex of five subsystems implemented by personal computers. The five subsystems are the communications front-end processor (CFEP), fax server, optical disk server, Document Capture Workstation (DCW), and magnetic disk server. The DRTS permits electronic document images to be stored temporarily (on magnetic disk) or permanently (on optical disk). The magnetic disk server provides access to documents stored on magnetic disk, and the optical disk server provides access to documents stored on optical disks. The magnetic disk server is a Novell NetWare-based computer with a Proteon 10MB/sec token ring network. Its primary function is to permit other computers in the network to share data and images. Though earlier studies showed that the size of a digitized and compressed page from a typical book in biomedicine scanned at 200dpi (dots per inch) was about 33KB,[3] most documents requested are likely to be journal articles. Being more tightly packed with text, images of journal pages yield a lower compression ratio resulting in image files roughly 70KB. With a storage size of a 300MB hard disk drive, the magnetic disk server permits temporary storage for approximately 9,000 biomedical book images or 4,200 journal page images.

The optical disk server permits access to documents stored on three Optimem 1,000 optical disk drives. Each drive houses a 12-inch optical disk platter that has a storage capacity of 2GB. This corresponds to a capacity of about 60,000 biomedical book images per platter.

The CFEP has two 2400-baud modems for answering incoming calls, and an interface to the token ring LAN. The CFEP provides an interface between remotely-located callers and the DRTS. With the two modems, it can handle two incoming calls simultaneously.

The fax server has an Intel SatisFAXtion board for faxing, a token ring LAN interface to the magnetic disk server, a Kofax image expansion board, and a laser printer. Its function is to fax documents or print them, depending on whether a user has requested the document to be transmitted by facsimile, to be mailed, or to be picked up.

The DCW serves the user who requests documents that are not stored online in electronic image form. It has an image compression/expansion board, and interfaces to a high-resolution (200dpi) charge coupled device (CCD) camera, 200dpi softcopy display device, and to the Novell Network-based magnetic disk server. It also has a local printer for printing a list of document requests for those documents that are not stored online. The DCW permits an operator to scan face-up bound volumes using the CCD camera. As each page of the document is scanned, its image appears on the softcopy display device, then is compressed and stored on the magnetic disk server. Another type of DCW recently developed incorporates a Fujitsu looseleaf page scanner that can scan at the rate of two seconds per page. This is ideal for unbound documents, and it automatically discriminates between the text and graphics portions of printed pages. While it does fixed-thresholding on textual sections, it dithers parts containing grayscale, such as photographs, to give them a better rendition when represented as bilevel digital images.

Functions

The functions of the EDDS subsystems are described below in more detail in order to explain the operation of the total system.

Document Request Workstation (DRW)

The design of the DRW is derived from prototype workstations previously designed for accessing image databases.[4,5] The DRW software presents the user with the following menu of functions:

1. Invoke GRATEFUL MED.
2. Choose Documents for Reception.
3. View/Modify Document List.
4. Call DRTS.
5. Run Setup.

Invoke GRATEFUL MED. With this option the user can run GRATEFUL MED, a user interface to MEDLINE, and several other databases on the NLM mainframe computer. It permits the user to enter search terms, then automatically calls the mainframe, logs in, does the search, downloads the search citations to a file on the local hard disk called the "output file," then logs off the mainframe. Back in Local mode, GRATEFUL MED permits the user to review the citations and formulate new search strategies without the expense of "staying on the line" connected to the mainframe.

Choose Documents for Reception. This option displays each citation one at a time from the output file created by GRATEFUL MED. For each citation, the user is asked whether the document is to be requested by fax, sent by mail, picked up by the user, or to do none of these. If the user chooses none, the next sequential citation is listed. If the user chooses fax, mail, or pickup, the software extracts the Unique Identifier (UI), author, and article title for this citation. The user may choose up to five citations.

View/Modify Document List. This option displays the documents requested by the user. It permits any request to be deleted, or method of transmission to be changed among the three methods: fax, mail, or pickup.

Call DRTS. When this option is invoked, the DRW creates a request file consisting of the user's name, facsimile telephone number, and a list of the chosen citations. It then calls the DRTS at the central document store. The CFEP answers the incoming calls and presents the user with a list of functions that are described in the CFEP section below.

Run Setup. This option permits a user to enter his/her name and facsimile telephone number, credit card information for billing purposes, plus address and the maximum amount the user is willing to pay per requested article. This information is sent with the document request file to the DRTS.

Communications Front-End Processor

Remote users who call the CFEP can do several things. They can submit orders for documents using citations selected from MEDLINE searches. They also can browse an online database of available documents and order documents directly from this database. Any document may be ordered to be delivered by facsimile transmission, mail, or pickup at the site of the DRTS. Finally, users can check on the status of previously-ordered documents. As requests for documents arrive, the CFEP inserts each request into a First-In-First-Out (FIFO) Request Queue on the magnetic disk server (see Figure 2). If the requested document exists online on optical disk, the request is then automatically routed to the optical disk server via a Request Queue. For documents that do not exist online, the request is routed to the DCW. The CFEP can handle two simultaneous incoming calls. At the time the CFEP answers a call, the file of up to five requested documents is automatically uploaded from the DRW to the CFEP. Each caller is then presented with a menu of functions:

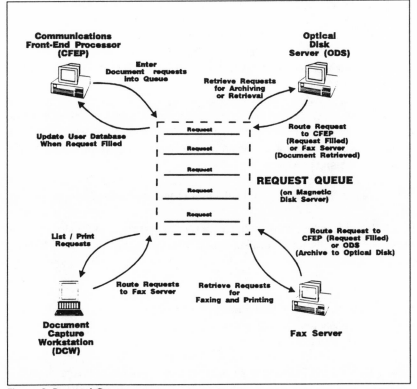

Figure 2. Request Queue

1. Browse Titles Available Online.
2. View All Document Requests.
3. Submit Document Requests.
4. Get Status on Orders.
5. Logout.

Browse Titles Available Online. The user may employ this option to view a list of documents that are available online for immediate transmission or mailing. For the case of journal articles, the user is first presented with a list of available journals. Once the user chooses a journal, the system lists all issues for that journal. On picking an issue, the user is presented with a list of articles in that issue. Then the user may select any article from this final list to be ordered. The user also selects the method of delivery at this time.

View All Document Requests. This option permits the user to view a list of documents requested either directly from the online browsing facility or by uploading requested documents during the call-in procedure. The user may delete any document from this list, or change the method of delivery.

Submit Document Requests. This option commands the CFEP to submit all requests for documents to the DRTS. These requests include those selected directly through the online browsing facility or via GRATEFUL MED searches uploaded during the call-in procedure.

Get Status on Orders. This option permits the user to receive the status on previously ordered documents. The status will indicate whether the document has been transmitted by facsimile, ready to be picked up, mailed, or the order is still being processed.

Logout. This option permits the user to log off the DRTS.

Besides the functions available for remote users, the CFEP also provides database functions for a local operator, who has a menu of the following choices:

1. Modify Cost.
2. View Billing Information.
3. Update the Browsing Index.
4. Go into Remote Mode.

Modify Cost. This option permits the local operator to change the dollar amount that requesters are to be charged for requested documents.

View Billing Information. The operator may use this option to view customer accounts to see which documents have been ordered, how many documents have been ordered, and how much they cost.

Update the Browsing Index. This option permits the operator to add new titles to the online browsing index.

Go into Remote Mode. This option allows the operator to set the CFEP into remote mode so that it can answer incoming calls.

Besides handling calls from remote users and operations invoked by the local operator, the CFEP also checks the Request Queue to handle document requests that have been filled (faxed or printed). These requests may be routed to the CFEP by either the fax server or optical disk server. It will be routed from the fax server for the case where a document on optical disk has been faxed or printed. It will be routed from the optical disk server for the case where a document newly created by the DCW has been faxed or printed, then archived to optical disk. For each completed request, the CFEP updates its user database to note that the request has been filled. This information is used in the CFEP's status function that tells users of the status of document orders.

Fax Server

The fax server fills document requests coming from DRWs. It does this by removing requests from the Request Queue. Requests for documents may be for facsimile transmission, mail, or pickup. Each document is accessed in the DRTS by a MEDLINE unique identifier. For each requested document, the fax server retrieves its images from the magnetic disk server, expands them from CCITT Group 4 compressed data, and converts them to DCX format, as required by the Intel SatisFAXtion board.[6] Both the magnetic disk server and optical disk server store images in Group 4 format, since this maximizes storage capacity. Images are expanded by the fax server using the image expansion board, then either printed on the laser printer or transmitted to the remote facsimile machines in Group 3 format by the SatisFAXtion board. It is necessary to convert from Group 4 to Group 3 format since current fax machines use the latter format. Once in CCITT Group 3 format, a document is transmitted to the requester's facsimile machine (if fax was requested). If the document is to be mailed to the requester or picked up at the central document store by the requester, the fax server skips the conversion to DCX format and instead prints the document on a local laser printer. After the transmission or printing is completed, the fax server checks to see if the document exists on optical disk. If it does, the fax server removes the document from magnetic disk and routes the document request to the CFEP. If the document does not exist on optical disk, the fax server sends the request to the optical disk server, which archives the document to optical disk.

Optical Disk Server

The optical disk server interfaces its three optical disk drives to the token ring network. It is responsible for retrieving document requests from the Request Queue that the CFEP has routed to it. For each request, the optical disk server transfers the correct document from optical disk to the magnetic disk server. Then it routes the request to the fax server, which in turn transmits or prints the document. The optical disk server also receives requests via the Request Queue from the fax server. Once the fax server finishes processing a document, it checks to see if the document exists on the optical disk server. The document will not exist there if it has been newly created by the DCW. Here, the optical disk server automatically archives the document to an optical disk, then routes the document request to the CFEP. By storing document images permanently on optical disk, the DRTS can automatically service requests for documents that are requested more than once, without requiring rescanning.

Document Capture Workstation

The DCW permits an operator to create electronic images of bound volumes and store them on the magnetic disk server. It has several functions for capturing, manipulating, and editing these document images. There are three subfunctions of interest to the discussion here:

1. Print Incoming Requests.
2. List Incoming Requests.
3. Create Request.

Print Incoming Requests. This function permits the operator of the DCW to obtain a printout of document requests in the Request Queue. Since these requests are for documents that are not stored online on either magnetic or optical disks in the DRTS, the printout of the requests is intended to allow a physical search of the local collection at the central document store. After a document is located, it may be brought to the DCW to be scanned.

List Incoming Requests. This option displays one request at a time on the computer monitor as each appears in the Request Queue. The screen shows all information about the document request, such as unique identifier, author, title, source, requester name, address, and facsimile telephone number. Once each request is displayed, the operator of the DCW may then scan the document pertaining to that request. After the document has been captured, the operator commands the DCW to send the document, and retrieve the next sequential request from the Request Queue. For each document to be sent, the DCW updates the entry for that document in the Request Queue, telling the fax server that the document is ready to be processed. The fax server, which periodically checks the Request Queue, senses this new status, then transmits or prints the document.

Create Request. This function permits a DCW operator to enter a document into the DRTS without a corresponding request coming to the fax server. This is intended to include requests that come from other sources, such as through the mail or by telephone. The Create Request function displays a form screen, into which the operator enters information about the document to be faxed or printed. Then the document is captured, and the request entered into the Request Queue, to be handled by the fax server.

EDDS as a Research Tool

The EDDS is a tool to address issues related to performance and cost, system design, and content selection. Among the issues that may be addressed using this prototype system as a testbed are the following:

- Does automated document delivery result in time and cost savings? By how much?
- What are the technical specifications of the hardware and software for an affordable automated document delivery system?
- What is the best user interface for the DRW? For the DCW? For the CFEP?
- What strategy should be used to select the part of the collection to be stored electronically? Are there subcollections better stored on magnetic disk (short-term storage) rather than optical disk (long-term storage)?
- What are alternative hardware architectures for the DCW? Should the DCW be portable? Should it be interfaced to the token ring network via radio transmission if it is portable? If a portable system is designed, what scanners, displays, and such, are best for integration into the DCW?
- What kinds of communications problems are encountered in an EDDS?
- How many users can be handled by the prototype implementation? What system design features facilitate migration to more users?

Status

As a result of comprehensive system testing, the current design of the EDDS has evolved and has undergone many improvements. The design described in this chapter is the third-generation EDDS. The DRTS in the first-generation EDDS consisted only of a fax server that handled one incoming call, a magnetic disk server, and an optical disk server. The second-generation system added the DCW to permit requests to be printed locally, and new documents to be scanned. The present system has also added automatic archiving to optical disk, and the CFEP with online title browsing, status facility, and capacity for two incoming calls. In addition, the DRTS permits additional DCWs, fax servers, CFEPs, or optical disk servers to be added to the system to accommodate higher throughput and document storage without any additional software modification. Both the first- and second-generation systems required the DRW to have an Intel SatisFAXtion for sending requests to the fax server. The present system eliminated this need, requiring the DRW to have just a Hayes-compatible modem. The user interface of the DRW has been redesigned to allow it to run on a laptop computer in addition to the present color monitor system. The third-generation EDDS is a suitable testbed to answer the key research questions.

References

1. R. Bharadwaj, "The Ariel Project," *Proc. ASIS*, vol. 28 (1991): 339.
2. National Network of Libraries of Medicine, Fact Sheet, National Library of Medicine, Bethesda MD 20894, June 1991.
3. F. L. Walker and G. R. Thoma, "Issues in archiving the medical literature with electronic imaging techniques," *Proceedings of Electronic Imaging '88 East*, Boston, Massachusetts, October 1988, pp. 590–95.
4. F. L. Walker and G. R. Thoma, "A hybrid system for retrieval of online biomedical citations and optical disk–based documents," *Proceedings of the Optical Publishing & Storage '87 Conference*, November 1987, pp. 179–91.
5. F. L. Walker and G. R. Thoma, "A prototype workstation for accessing and using an optical disk–based database of biomedical documents," *Proceedings of the 1989 ASIS Mid-Year Meeting*, San Diego, CA, May 1989.
6. *The DCA/Intel Communicating Applications Specification*, Version 1.0A, Digital Communications Associates, Inc., and Intel Corporation, September 1988.

CHAPTER 8.
FULL-TEXT DIGITIZED IMAGES: A COLLABORATIVE PROJECT BETWEEN SCIENTIFIC PUBLISHERS, PHYSICIANS, COMPUTER EXPERTS, AND LIBRARIANS.

Jeffrey S. Hylton
Assistant Director Technology and
Communications Systems
Georgetown University Medical Center

Naomi C. Broering
Director, Biomedical Information Resources Center
and Medical Center Librarian
Georgetown University Medical Center
Dahlgren Memorial Library

Helen E. Bagdoyan
Associate Librarian for Planning and
Database Development
Georgetown University Medical Center

Abstract

The Dahlgren Memorial Library at Georgetown University has undertaken an experimental project to digitize the full text of articles from selected genetic and cancer journals. The project, called a Digital Full-Text Biotechnology System, is an electronic full-text database created from scanned images of journal article pages which include both text and illustrations. The Digital Full-Text Biotechnology System will be linked to the Library's existing bibliographic search systems such as the miniMEDLINE SYSTEM™ and ALERTS™/Current Contents®. The project will provide online, fax, and mail access to the digitized articles. A working prototype provides the basic functions of searching, retrieving, and display of the articles.

Introduction

Medical libraries have traditionally provided services that include biblio-graphic searches and access to current medical and scientific journals. Tech-nological advances over the last fifteen years have significantly increased the breadth of the searches possible and reduced the amount of time required to retrieve relevant biomedical information. The end result usually entails deliv-ery of a paper document to the library patron. Computers and document de-livery software have also provided a convenient and coordinated electronic ordering and tracking system for procuring documents from within and out of the local library. Some computer vendors provide online access to full text such as legal systems and limited journals. These systems provide only computer printouts and do not include illustrations.

Today, however, the technology exists to display pictures, graphs, and charts along with text of an article. This additional information is often critical for the scientific researcher who relies heavily on the illustrations and charts accompanying the text of articles. The Dahlgren Memorial Library at George-town University has undertaken an experimental project, funded by a grant from the U.S. Department of Education, to provide patrons with full-text arti-cles from selected journals complete with illustrations. The Digital Full-Text Biotechnology System will augment the Library's existing bibliographic search systems with digitized images of each page in selected journals.

Collaboration between publishers, physicians, researchers, computer experts, and librarians has been carefully executed because it is essential for development of a quality system that meets the needs of the modern healthcare professional. Advisory committees have been formulated to provide expert advice for steering the project forward (see Figure 1).

Overview

The Georgetown University™ Library Information System (LIS) includes an integrated Document Delivery System (DDS). Today, library patrons can search the miniMEDLINE SYSTEM™ and ALERTS™/Current Contents® bibliographic systems and electronically request documents from successful searches. The electronic requests for in-house material are automatically routed to photocopy services. Requests for documents outside the library are routed to interlibrary loan services (ILL). The patron can request journal articles to be delivered by fax, mail, or pick-up at the library. For journals that are owned by the library, a staff member will find the correct journal, photocopy the article, and then transmit it over fax, mail, or set it aside for pickup.

An electronic database of the full text of journal articles will automate this process by significantly accelerating and simplifying delivery to users.

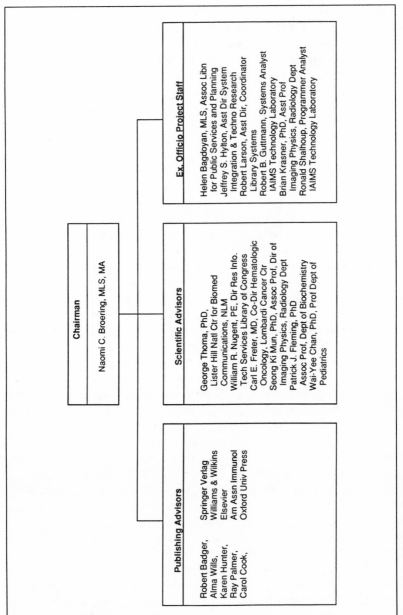

Figure 1. Advisory Committees

Once scanned and stored, the articles can be printed, faxed, or viewed on a computer screen without the time-consuming process of finding the journal and photocopying. For example, an article can be retrieved from the database and automatically faxed without the need for a paper copy. If a paper copy is needed for mailing, the digital image of each page of the article is retrieved from the electronic database and routed to a laser printer without the need to locate the original paper copy of the journal.

In addition to the library's digital journal print and fax functions, patrons will have the capability of viewing the full text as well as the illustrations and graphics of an article directly at the search workstation. This is a powerful tool that immediately puts the contents of an article in the hands of a physician or researcher. Busy doctors often do not have time to walk to the library to find a journal. Even an Online Public Access Catalog (OPAC) cannot predict whether the specific journal will actually be on the shelf or in use, perhaps in a study carrel. Digitizing the articles also creates a library that never sleeps and is never too busy or understaffed to find and fax an article immediately. A digital full-text storage and retrieval system will help meet the growing need to provide information beyond the physical walls of the library.

The development of a prototypic digital full-text biotechnology system provides the Dahlgren Library with a tool for exploring the technology of storing and transmitting full-text documents. The design of the system is robust enough to potentially expand the database to include images that can be linked to systems outside the sphere of bibliographic search systems. Possibilities include links to the OPAC for displaying images of medical illustrations or pictures of historical items in the Library's collection. There are a myriad of possible applications once an image database and retrieval method is created.

There are several off-the-shelf software packages available today that provide the ability to combine full-text and keyword searching with image retrieval. These products cover a broad range of costs and capabilities. Many of the vendor products are sold as "document management" systems. They are designed for the business or office environment to manage, track, and retrieve documents more quickly than relying on paper copies in filing cabinets. All provide some sort of search mechanism, whether based on keywords or the indexed words of the full text. Some vendors have started to provide support for multiple hardware platforms. Unfortunately, many document management systems are closed systems that only support a specific hardware platform such as the Apple Macintosh or 80x86 personal computers, but not both.[1]

Developing a digital full-text retrieval system in-house has some distinct advantages over the off-the-shelf products. The main advantage is the ability to integrate the new system with the existing bibliographic search systems which are already in place and familiar to the library patrons. The miniMEDLINE SYSTEM has been in use at Georgetown since 1981. It is an in-house subset of the MEDLINE files developed by the National Library of Medicine (NLM). The miniMEDLINE SYSTEM has a powerful bibliographic retrieval system that is extremely easy to use. The database is searchable by journal name, title word, author, and Medical Subject Heading (MeSH term). This in-house database spans five years and contains references and abstracts to 1,100 journal titles received by the Library which are indexed in the NLM's MED-LINE database. The system is updated monthly. It is heavily used; over 31,000 miniMEDLINE search sessions were conducted by users in 1991.

ALERTS/Current Contents is similar to the miniMEDLINE SYSTEM except that it contains references and abstracts to journal articles contained in the Institute for Scientific Information's (ISI) Current Contents system. This system is updated weekly and provides up-to-date information on publications since the articles included are not yet indexed by the NLM or other database developers. In 1991, library patrons used the system over 5,000 times. Linking the miniMEDLINE and ALERTS/Current Contents systems to a database of digitized journals articles puts a powerful tool in the hands of healthcare professionals without forcing them to relearn a new system or sacrifice the proven search capabilities of miniMEDLINE and ALERTS/Current Contents.

What the Researcher Sees

The researcher sits down at a special workstation (initially a Sun SPARCstation) and connects to the Dahlgren Library's Knowledge Network. The Knowledge Network provides access to a family of databases including bibliographic, informational, factual, diagnostic, and e-mail systems. In this case, the user will access the bibliographic systems to search miniMEDLINE or ALERTS/Current Contents. After entering search terms (e.g., John Smith, lymphoma) and combining search sets with the proper Boolean operators, the researcher reviews the resulting literature references. Most references have abstracts that can be read online and miniMEDLINE also displays the associated MeSH terms. If the full text of the article is also available, a prompt asks if the patron wishes to view the article. The article is then displayed in a new pop-up window on the screen (see Figure 2). The scientist will be able to scroll up and down, move between pages, zoom in on graphs or illustrations to see specific details, or print it to a locally connected laser printer. After viewing the document, the full-text window will disappear and searching can be continued in miniMEDLINE. If the article needs to be printed, faxed, or mailed, the researcher can press D for Document Delivery and the fax/photocopy/ILL services are available online.

The search interface is identical for patrons who are not using a special graphics workstation, except that there will not be a prompt for full text nor will a window with the text image pop up. Today, scientists and physicians at Georgetown can access the Library's computer resources from the office, lab, home, library public workstations, and even from their coworker's offices. The

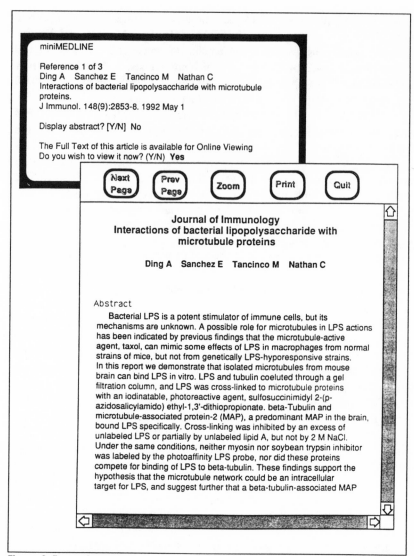

miniMEDLINE

Reference 1 of 3
Ding A   Sanchez E   Tancinco M   Nathan C
Interactions of bacterial lipopolysaccharide with microtubule
proteins.
J Immunol. 148(9):2853-8. 1992 May 1

Display abstract? [Y/N] No

The Full Text of this article is available for Online Viewing
Do you wish to view it now? (Y/N) **Yes**

Next Page   Prev Page   Zoom   Print   Quit

Journal of Immunology
Interactions of bacterial lipopolysaccharide with
microtubule proteins

Ding A   Sanchez E   Tancinco M   Nathan C

Abstract
    Bacterial LPS is a potent stimulator of immune cells, but its
mechanisms are unknown. A possible role for microtubules in LPS actions
has been indicated by previous findings that the microtubule-active
agent, taxol, can mimic some effects of LPS in macrophages from normal
strains of mice, but not from genetically LPS-hyporesponsive strains.
In this report we demonstrate that isolated microtubules from mouse
brain can bind LPS in vitro. LPS and tubulin coeluted through a gel
filtration column, and LPS was cross-linked to microtubule proteins
with an iodinatable, photoreactive agent, sulfosuccinimidyl 2-(p-
azidosalicylamido) ethyl-1,3'-dithiopropionate. beta-Tubulin and
microtubule-associated protein-2 (MAP), a predominant MAP in the brain,
bound LPS specifically. Cross-linking was inhibited by an excess of
unlabeled LPS or partially by unlabeled lipid A, but not by 2 M NaCl.
Under the same conditions, neither myosin nor soybean trypsin inhibitor
was labeled by the photoaffinity LPS probe, nor did these proteins
compete for binding of LPS to beta-tubulin. These findings support the
hypothesis that the microtubule network could be an intracellular
target for LPS, and suggest further that a beta-tubulin-associated MAP

Figure 2. Example screens

ability to integrate full text into the universally accessible miniMEDLINE and
ALERTS/Current Contents provides much more continuity than a stand-alone
vendor package that is only available to certain types of workstations in designated locations with specific user codes. While initially users without a special workstation will not be able to view the full text of the articles online, they

will still get the benefits of the electronic full-text database when requesting a fax or printout of the articles via the DDS. Plans are to develop the view capability on other workstations in phase two of the project.

How the System Works

Specially modified software on the Sun SPARCstation provides the patron with a VT-100 character-based terminal emulator (see Figure 3). A connection is made to the Knowledge Network via either the campus-wide AT&T ISN asynchronous communications network or the Ethernet-based High-Speed Network (HSN). After selecting miniMEDLINE from the menu, a session is established with the DEC VAX 8550 running miniMEDLINE. While displaying the selected citations, miniMEDLINE checks an index to determine if the article is contained in the full-text database. If so, a library unique identifier (LUI) (rhymes with gooey) is sent back to the SPARCstation that uniquely identifies the article. A program is called on the workstation that connects to an image server. The program retrieves the article and displays it in a new window.

When a patron uses the DDS for print or fax requests of online full-text articles, DDS sends the request to a special print server or fax server instead of the normal human-to-stacks-to-photocopy route. The print and fax servers request the digitized document from the image server and then handle the distribution electronically. Once entered into the Digital Full-Text Biotechnology System database, a library staff member no longer needs to track down and photocopy a specific journal. Everything, except actually reading the article, is performed electronically.

The image server software resides on a Sun SPARCserver. This software provides full-text image workstations and other future client applications with a standard set of instructions for retrieving images. The software under development at Georgetown has not been purchased from a vendor for three main reasons.

1. Vendor systems are much more difficult to integrate with the existing in-house bibliographic search systems.
2. The retrieval programs can be distributed to client workstations without licensing problems and expense of vendor-supplied client workstation software (e.g., some SQL client software costs more than $200 per workstation).
3. The generic retrieval instructions will be independent of the actual method used to store the images. This separation of the retrieval function from the database storage function allows the database to remain independent from the client retrieval software.

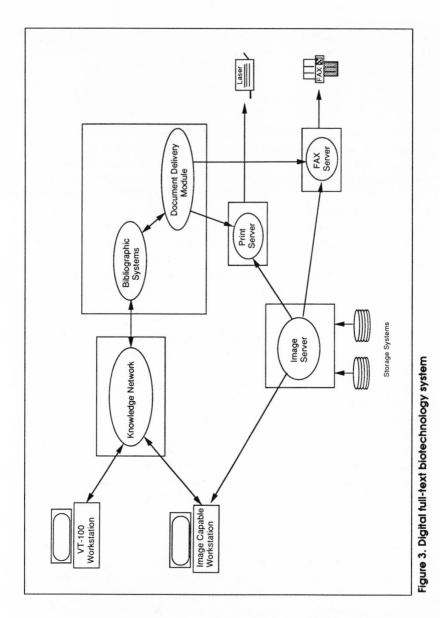

Figure 3. Digital full-text biotechnology system

Only part of the server software needs to be updated if the images are moved from one storage method to another. A single image server provides a link to the images wherever they may reside in the future.

The Full-Text Database

Since the project is experimental in nature, a large database of journals is not initially required to test the technical aspects of the system. Ten journals were selected to start the project. An advisory committee which includes representatives from several publishing companies have reviewed and selected the titles. They have recommended expanding the journals in the initial database and this is being considered. Georgetown is heavily committed to research in the field of biotechnology. To support these endeavors and to fill unmet information needs, the digitized full-text project will focus on journals in the fields of cancer and genetics. The Lombardi Cancer Research Institute, the Department of Pediatrics, the AIDS Virology Project in the Department of Microbiology and several basic science departments will benefit directly from the first-known full-text document delivery system dedicated to cancer and genetics journals.

The articles will be scanned using a high-speed scanner. The image database will consist of black and white images saved in the TIFF format and compressed using the Consultative Committee on International Telegraphy and Telephony (CCITT) Group 4 compression algorithm. During an initial testing period, the best scanner settings will be determined for the text in each journal. Factors such as font type and size, the darkness of the characters, and the type and thickness of paper will all influence the settings for obtaining optimal readability of the digital article. Once the settings are known for each journal, experimentation will not be required until a new journal issue arrives. Unfortunately, nearly all pictures and many of the illustrations and charts within the articles may have to be rescanned with different settings to maximize their clarity. Text and illustrations usually require different settings and it is best to scan a page multiple times and combine the clearest images of both text and illustrations rather than use a compromise setting that creates an unsatisfactory image of both. A good example of this problem can be seen in a typical photocopy of an article with a picture on it. Even the best exposure setting copies the text with a black unrecognizable picture.

The cut-and-paste method will provide the best quality image for each page of an article but it comes at a significant cost in labor. The ten journals selected contain approximately 40,000 pages per year. In order to reduce the enormous manpower involved in scanning, cutting, and pasting the articles, an automated method of creating the best image of both the text and graphics from a single scan is being considered. This method involves scanning the pages as 8-bit gray-scale images instead of 1-bit black and white images and then running one or more special image enhancement programs on the images to enhance the text. The gray-scale image is then converted to black and white for inclusion in the image database. Although the resultant image is not quite as good as the cut-and-paste method, it offers significant savings in staff time.

The resolution of the scanning is equally important and must be considered when creating an image database. Images are scanned and displayed at a certain number of dots per inch (dpi). The higher the resolution, the crisper the image and the bigger the file. The articles for this project will be scanned at 300dpi. At 200dpi, the resolution used by fax machines, would probably be sufficient for the immediate returns expected from the printing and faxing aspects of the project. However, the higher resolution of the 300dpi images will not only provide better displays when interactively zooming in on certain parts of an article page, but it also captures detail from the article that would otherwise be lost if scanned at the lower resolution. There is no way to recover information lost from scanning at a lower resolution when a higher resolution is needed later. The 300dpi scan will provide an accurate image in a reasonable amount of disk space. Forthcoming software and hardware available for printing and faxing will be able to take advantage of the 300dpi resolution to produce better output. The additional resolution will also be needed in the future if and when the images are submitted to optical character recognition (OCR) software. These programs require the higher resolution in order to convert the image of the page into ASCII text.

There are many different file formats available for storing images. Nearly each "paint" package uses a different format for storing and reading images. Generally, in order for different computers to view an image it must be stored separately for each package or a special program is needed to convert the file to a format known to the package before loading. Viewing software for each of the intended types of full-text workstations (MAC, PC, SPARC) will be written that can use a common image file format. A single format is required to prevent duplication of images in the database and/or eliminate the delay and CPU overhead of converting the file each time it is displayed. The Tagged Image File Format (TIFF) has been chosen because it is a flexible format and is supported by many software packages across different hardware platforms. The TIFF image files will be compressed using the CCITT Group 4 (G4) algorithm. The G4 has been selected as the compression technique because it offers significant image compression and is becoming a standard for storing black and white images similar to those used in this project. The G4 offers significant compression ratios that exceed the CCITT Group 3 (G3) format that is currently used in standard fax machines.[2] Exact compression ratios vary by individual image and the method of comparison, but compression of 20:1 or 30:1 are possible.

A single page scanned at 300dpi will take up approximately a megabyte of storage space when scanned and stored in TIFF format. The CCITT Group 4 file compression format is more efficient for storing black and white images and therefore takes up less space. The storage requirements can be reduced to as little as 40 kilobytes for each article page (50 to 100K per page may be more likely depending on the scanning technique used and the quality of the original journal article). The smaller files require less disk storage and also less time to transmit across a network. The full-text image project is network based and transmission time is directly related to the size of the page image. In a multi-workstation environment, a large number of simultaneous article retrievals could cripple a server and the network if all of the images are stored and transmitted at their full size.

The Prototype System: Phase I

A working prototype of the full-text image system has been created. A working model provides a testbed for networking issues as well as conceptual design. The modules which deal with identification of the article, retrieval, and display the digital images of the article pages have been prototyped and linked together into a test system. The prototype has been demonstrated and discussed with various people including technical advisors and representatives from publishing companies. The response has been very positive.

The full-text biotechnology system is made up of nine distinct modules which interact to form the complete system. The modules are:

1. modified VT-100 emulation software;
2. enhanced miniMEDLINE and ALERTS/Current Contents software;
3. image server database;
4. image retrieval software;
5. decompression/view software;
6. image database/bibliographic index maintenance;
7. image scan/edit/view/conversion/compression workstation;
8. fax full-text articles; and
9. print full-text articles.

VT-100 Emulation

The current miniMEDLINE software uses a character-based user interface with menus to lead users through a search. Character-based applications at Georgetown University generally use the screen control sequences used by the Digital Equipment Corporation (DEC) VT series of terminals. The mini-MEDLINE and ALERTS/Current Contents systems follow the Georgetown standard by formatting the screen using VT-100 screen calls. There are many different sources for terminal emulation software that will allow a IBM PC (or clone), an Apple MAC, or X-Window workstation to mimic the original VT-100 hardware.

The initial user workstation for the prototype is a Sun SPARCstation IPC. The public domain programs XVT TOOL and VTEM provide a VT-100 emulator for the X-Window environment and the basic interface to miniMEDLINE and ALERTS. Modifications were made to the underlaying VTEM software so that the SPARCstation can identify itself to the bibliographic search software (module 2) as a "special image capable" VT-100 workstation and receive an image's LUI and pass it to the image retrieval software (module 4).

Enhanced miniMEDLINE and ALERTS/Current Contents Software

Several enhancements were made to the bibliographic software including:

- a new index file structure to identify articles that are in the digital full-text database;
- special codes, sent out at the beginning of the miniMEDLINE or ALERTS session workstation to determine if it is "image capable"; and
- a new program to inform the user that the full text of the selected article is available online then transmit its LUI to the workstation.

The changes to the document delivery software which will route print or fax requests to the appropriate electronic full-text biotechnology modules instead of routing them to the normal human channel are in progress.

Image Server/Database

The heart of the entire system is the actual image database module. This module provides storage for the images as well as an image server which takes requests for the images, retrieves them from the database, and transmits them back to the client workstation (module 4).

The images are stored as raw files on the Sun SPARCserver's disk drives. A special indexed file contains pointers to the images as well as important information such as the number of pages in the article, the size of the images, and the location of the images files on the disk drives. The prototype uses the Wide Area Information Server (WAIS) software from Thinking Machines Inc., as the front end to the image database. This software is in the public domain and provides a client/server environment where multiple types of workstations can query and retrieve information from the central database.[3] It was easily adapted to use the library's indexed database file instead of the native WAIS format.

As the project progresses, the images may be transferred from the current storage method to an SQL database like Sybase. The Dahlgren Library currently uses Sybase for in-house systems such as Faculty Publications Online and Medical Facts File. Sybase provides good management tools which may help reduce the maintenance and labor costs as the image database grows. SQL can also provide another client/server access method to the image database for future projects.

The current prototype database is very small and therefore the storage requirements are also small. A full production system is expected to grow rapidly and have immense storage requirements. Standard magnetic hard disks and optical media have both been investigated for storing the images. Optical drives offer a cost per megabyte savings over the magnetic drives,[4] however, the recent drop in costs of magnetic drives plus their significantly faster retrieval speed makes them the preferred approach.

Image Retrieval Software

The image retrieval module consists of software that resides on the user's workstation. It functions to link the user's workstation via the ethernet to the image server (module 3) and request an article using the LUI for identification. The resultant images are transferred to the user's workstation organized in such a way that the decompression/viewing software (module 5) can access them easily.

The prototype uses a combination of shell scripts and WAIS retrieval software to download the article pages. WAIS provides an excellent method for transferring both image and text files across the network.

Decompression/View Software

The software will display the full-text images of the selected article in a new window at the user's workstation. Since the images will be transferred in a compressed format, the file will have to be decompressed prior to loading it into the new viewer window. The 300dpi resolution of the image will create a picture far larger than the workstation's screen (typically 70 to 100dpi). The view software will scale the image to fit the window and provide a mechanism for moving page to page. Users will also need to be able to zoom in on parts of the image in order to see more detail on charts and illustrations.

The prototype currently uses files in the native Sun raster format instead of the TIFF format. The current viewer is simple and does not have advanced features such as zooming.

Image Database/Bibliographic Index Maintenance

As the journals are published and received by the Library, a report will be run to create a list of the articles for that journal issue as they are indexed in

ALERTS/Current Contents and miniMEDLINE. Each article will be listed with its assigned LUI. When the articles are scanned (module 7), the staff person running the scanner will save the article using the assigned LUI.

Each article will be transferred to a loading directory on the image server. The indexing programs will take the files for each article and load them into the image database. The index files in the image database as well as the index files in the miniMEDLINE and ALERTS/Current Contents systems will also be updated automatically so that the article can be retrieved.

Image Scan/Edit/View/Conversion/Compression Workstation

A special scanning workstation is designated to incorporate a high-speed black and white scanner, scanning software, image edit software, a high-resolution monitor, image conversion and compression software, and access to the Ethernet network.

To scan the articles ideally, the spines of the journals would be cut off. This provides individual sheets of paper that can be quickly fed through the sheet feeder of the scanner. Since journals are valuable resources to a library (even if available electronically), unless duplicate copies are available this procedure will not be used for all journals in the project.

The exact method for obtaining the best image of both the text and the graphics is still being investigated. Regardless of whether the cut-and-paste or the software enhancement method is used, the final image will be converted to the TIFF format and then compressed. The images for each article would be assigned the proper LUI (module 6) and transferred via the Ethernet to the load directory on the image server for processing and indexing into the image database.

FAX Full-Text Articles

A special fax server program running on the Sun SPARCstation will accept an article LUI and fax number from the Document Delivery Module of the Library Information System (LIS). The associated electronic article will be requested from the image server and then the article will be sent to the library patron using a special fax card attached to the computer.

Since the articles in the database are always online, the patron will not have to wait until a staff member is free to search the stacks, photocopy, and then place the article in a fax machine. The library patron will receive faster service for the full text of these articles.

Print Full-Text Articles

This software is very similar to the fax software described above. A program running on a SPARCstation will accept an article LUI from the LIS

Document Delivery Module. The electronic article will be printed out on a laser printer located in the Library for pickup or mailing.

Project Status

The current prototype solidly provides modules 1 through 4 from the list above. Some parts of modules 5, 6, 7, and 9 are also complete. The fax module relies on special hardware and software that has not arrived yet.

The work reported here is still in prototype form. Although the prototype provides a working model, some modules are not fully integrated. The modular approach offers definite advantages. Each module in the full-text biotechnology system performs a certain function that is distinct, and can therefore can be enhanced and replaced as needed without affecting the functionality of the system as a whole. The prototype modules will be replaced as needed one at a time. The modular construction of the prototype allows an easy migration path upwards from the current test system towards a final production system.

Statistics will be maintained at several places within the modules to track the usage of the system. The data will help the Library study how the electronic full-text of articles is used when it is made available to library patrons. The collaborative arrangement between libraries, scientists, and publishers will hopefully provide a fertile model for future cooperative endeavors and research activities.

References

1. *Choosing the Right Imaging System* (Micro Dynamics, Ltd.: Silver Spring, MD, 1990).
2. P. J. Latimer, "Binary vs. grayscale images: a tradeoff of storage vs. quality," *Imaging* 1 (July 1992): 20–23.
3. B. Kahle and A. Medlar, "An information system for corporate users: Wide Area Information Servers," *Online* 15 (September 1991): 56–60.
4. R. Wilson, "Rewriteable optical." *SunWorld* 4 (June 1991): 72–80.

Bibliographic References

Thoma, G. R. and F. L. Walker. A Prototype Electronic Document Delivery System. *ASIS 90: Proceedings of the 53rd ASIS Annual Meeting,* 1990 November 4–8, Toronto, Ontario. Diane Henderson et al., eds. (Medford, NJ: Learned Information, 1990), 29–35.

Wilson, D. L. "Major scholarly publisher to test electronic transmission of journals." *The Chronical of Higher Education* (June 3, 1992): A17–A20.

CHAPTER 9.
MEDICAL INFORMATION MANAGEMENT AND LIBRARIES: THE EXTENDED ONLINE CATALOG

Helen E. Bagdoyan
*Associate Librarian for Planning and
Database Development
Georgetown University Medical Center*

Abstract

As electronic information resources become more plentiful and user demands for information continue to escalate, libraries with the most advanced catalogs will have the ability to link users into a "global library." The advanced catalog becomes the extended online catalog and possesses features such as true authority control, powerful searching capabilities, links to other files, and access to external networks. Foundations for the extended online catalog began in the 1970s and 1980s with the development of integrated library systems and medical libraries have been at the cutting edge of this development from the start. The first priority was bibliographic control, and the second, access to the content of the biomedical knowledge base. Horizons in the 1990s focus on national networks, intelligent retrieval capabilities, and digitized images. The Georgetown University Medical Center Library has been in the forefront of library automation and database development. The evolution of its Knowledge Network and the wide range of over twenty databases, bibliographic and beyond, are described in this chapter.

Introduction

Knowledge is of two kinds: we know a subject ourselves or we know where we can find information upon it.[1]

Samuel Johnson, 1709–84

The concept of an extended online catalog conveys an ability to go beyond the usual limits. The old card catalog, and even the single-function online catalog, implied limitations: a particular library, collection, or resource. With advanced computer and communications technology and the development of integrated library systems, the extended online catalog is evolving gradually into a "global library."

To the scholar, physician, scientist, and student in the biomedical disciplines, the extended online catalog evokes positive images:

- unlimited access to multiple information resources;
- elimination of time, location, ownership, and format as barriers to information transfer and exchange; and
- an expansion into new realms of information creation and management.

To the library and information science professional who provides access to the content of biomedical resources, the environment of an extended online catalog presents opportunities to:

- broaden the biomedical knowledge base;
- shift emphasis from ownership to access;
- encourage resource sharing; and
- distribute costs for expensive resources among many.

This chapter defines the extended online catalog by describing the foundations from which the extended online catalog emerged in the early 1980s and tracing its continued evolution and enhancements into the 1990s. Attention is directed to the role of medical libraries as major players in the development of integrated library systems and how, in the 1980s, these pioneering libraries virtually redefined the online catalog. Trends in the 1990s are bringing additional changes to the extended online catalog with new methods of access through national networks and the design of intelligent retrieval capabilities to navigate users invisibly in searching multiple databases. The sections entitled "Building the Knowledge Network" and "Databases at the Cutting Edge" focus on the experience at Georgetown in implementing a medical decision-support system. The chapter provides descriptive details on the range of databases available for use by health professionals in education, research, and patient care.

The Extended Online Catalog Defined

The existence of an online catalog takes many forms. Its characteristics surpass the confines of the traditional catalog and its potential for adaptation and change have never been more evident than it is today. Prior to 1980, the design of online catalogs concentrated on the replication of the card catalog with the intent of recycling an existing tool into an electronic environment. Culkin considers the word catalog to be too conservative. "It has a finite connotation: its bounds are drawn by the holdings of the library. The word itself limits and perhaps even prevents creative thinking about how the resource can be developed to its fullest . . . potential."[2] According to Hildreth, "the online catalog will never be a finished, perfected project . . . Today's online catalog stands apart from earlier catalogs because it is interactive, infinitely expandable, and public."[3]

In the mid- to late 1980s, a number of authors elaborated on the next generation of library automation systems and predicted great potential and profound changes ahead for public access computer systems.[4,5,6,7] Jaffee saw a new career for the online catalog, with a proliferation of features for the information user that includes printing, downloading, remote access, gateways, user interfaces, and supercatalogs.[8] As single-function systems evolve into integrated systems, the user is provided with a single source, a common interface, and a unified environment in which to retrieve information, according to Potter.[9] By consensus, the most advanced catalogs—the extended online catalogs—have true authority control, powerful searching capabilities, linkages to other files, and access to external networks.

Innovations by Medical Libraries in the 1980s

The foundation for the extended online catalog was based on the development of integrated library systems. In the late 1970s and early 1980s, medical libraries, such as the National Library of Medicine (NLM), the Israel National Library, Washington University, and Georgetown University, undertook pioneering efforts in the design and implementation of totally integrated library systems.[10,11,12,13,14,15]

Several developers and users of integrated systems shared similar visions of what an integrated library system should provide in its initial stages and in its future capabilities.[16,17,18,19] Two key concepts were stressed and centered on control and access. Control is achieved in the automation of basic library functions (cataloging, circulation, serials control, acquisitions) in an integrated approach with provisions for individual components to share and exchange information. The second concept, access, focuses on providing users with direct access and retrieval of information that goes beyond the bibliographic reference into the actual contents of articles and books, into full-text, numeric, and factual information, and into graphic representations. In addition, the importance of users being able to find needed information themselves from multiple resources within the library's collections and from external sources was widely recognized.

Several pioneering libraries in the field of automation designed and implemented value-added components to their integrated library systems.[20,21,22,23,24,25] Once these libraries stepped beyond the operational functions into value-added software development, the concept of an extended online catalog emerged. The ability to go beyond the bibliographic reference into the actual information content became a reality and set the stage for the extended online catalog with each library defining the breadth of its own catalog based on user needs and the institutional mission.

In reviewing the successful automation projects of the 1980s, the major accomplishments for that decade were the development of integrated library systems, the proliferation of, and access to, databases that go beyond the online catalog, and the ability to access systems locally and from remote sites.

New Directions for the 1990s

Interest in the 1990s continues to stress the development of databases and the enhanced integration of library systems. The big thrusts in automation, however, are concentrating on newer directions, such as national networking capabilities, intelligent user interfaces, and the access and transmission of digitized images.

Networks

Online access through national networks, such as the Internet, provides an opportunity for libraries and information users to tap into resources not available at their own institutions. High-speed networks, advanced communications technology, and accessibility of shared databases is making it possible for any user at any workstation to find needed information. The end result is a payoff with equal advantages to information users and providers, as envisioned in the following scenario:

> It is after midnight. A patient at an inner-city hospital goes into crisis and presents with unusual symptoms The medical resident on duty acts quickly to handle the patient's immediate care and then begins to plan for longer term management. The usual channels of information-gathering are not available at this late hour. The medical library is closed; colleagues are not at the hospital. The resident has other choices, however, because his institution has online information resources available at workstations close to patient sites. At the nearest workstation, the resident taps into several online databases, in rapid succession, to formulate plans for managing the critical patient at-hand. He uses a drug information system, several literature databases, and a file of full-text articles. What he does not know is that none of the databases he uses this evening are located at his institution. He has tapped into a system of

"shared resources" created by a consortium of libraries that are geographically dispersed throughout the United States. Access is made possible through the Internet with a communications protocol that guides him invisibly from one geographic area to another, wherever the particular information resource is located. The drug system, initial literature databases, and full-text files are at Georgetown University in Washington, D.C. The full MEDLINE database is at Rush University in Chicago. The resident is at a university hospital in Lubbock, Texas. Multiple institutions, in a consortial arrangement, are sharing their unique information resources to broaden the knowledge base available to their combined constitutents. Shrinking budgets have compelled libraries to develop consortial projects for resource sharing and technology has made it possible to share these resources electronically.

Intelligent Retrieval Capabilities

With the enormous proliferation of databases, the bewildered information seeker needs assistance to navigate through the maze of systems, and several projects are underway to develop software with intelligent retrieval capabilities. These include the Unified Medical Language System™ (UMLS®), the GRATEFUL MED® software for searching NLM databases, and Georgetown's BioSYNTHESIS project.

UMLS. Sponsored by the NLM, UMLS is designed to facilitate the retrieval and integration of information from multiple machine-readable biomedical information sources, such as the literature, clinical records, databanks, knowledge-based systems, and directories of people and organizations. The variety of vocabularies and classifications used in different sources is a significant barrier to the use of machine-readable databases by health professionals and biomedical researchers. The UMLS approach assumes continued diversity in the terminology employed in different systems and by users themselves and concentrates on the development of effective search interfaces to assist users.[26]

GRATEFUL MED. GRATEFUL MED software is a front-end program designed to simplify the process of searching the NLM databases, such as MEDLINE. GRATEFUL MED helps formulate a search, connects to the NLM computer, runs the search, disconnects from the NLM computer, and displays/prints/downloads search results.

BioSYNTHESIS. This is a prototype intelligent retrieval system under development at Georgetown. The purpose is to create an integrated system that can retrieve information from multiple in-house and external databases from a single point of entry. BioSYNTHESIS I involved the design of a single menu to access various databases that reside on different computers. BioSYNTHESIS II is an ongoing research project concerned with the development of a search component that facilitates complex searching. Its purpose is to navigate the user in a transparent manner and provide access to multiple databases.[27, 28, 29]

Building the Knowledge Network

Georgetown has created a prototype Knowledge Network of core information resources that are scattered throughout the Medical Center (and beyond), brought them together into one electronic system, and offers Georgetown users access free of charge. This has been accomplished from a foundation established in the early 1980s with the implementation of the Georgetown University™ Library Information System (LIS) and its family of bibliographic databases. Expansion of the network occurred throughout the 1980s with the informational, diagnostic, and factual database development projects implemented through the Integrated Advanced Information Management System (IAIMS) program. Continued enhancements, underway in the 1990s, feature new database development projects, such as storage and retrieval of full-text documents and digitizing images for access and transmission.

At Georgetown, both LIS and IAIMS helped to wake the sleeping giant of the 1980's "information decade." These succesful automation projects have exerted considerable influence to change the way health professionals access information. Every facet of healthcare delivery, education, and research at the Georgetown University Medical Center has been affected by the advances made in the automation and integration of information resources. This is evident in the way physicians and nurses care for patients on a daily basis, how health professions students are taught and what they learn, which databanks are in high demand by bench scientists, the variety and complexity of information resources provided by the library, and the manner in which the Medical Center's major computer systems link and share information.

Georgetown has been able to develop its innovative Knowledge Network in an evolutionary manner. From the beginning, the basic system architecture of LIS was planned so that a total information environment could evolve. The Medical Library's Online Catalog was introduced in 1981. The real milestone, however, to mark the birth of Georgetown's extended online catalog occurred in 1982, when the miniMEDLINE SYSTEM™ was introduced.[30] The introduction of miniMEDLINE, one of the first end-user databases for searching the content of journal articles, was a pivotal point in the evolutionary process that produced the Georgetown Knowledge Network. From 1981 to the present, this network has grown in depth and scope, and today, users can select from a wide range of databases. The chronology outlined in Table 1 emphasizes this gradual growth.

TABLE 1. Georgetown Knowledge Network: Database Implementation	
1981 Online Catalog	**1989** Molecular Biology
1982 miniMEDLINE **1986** Alerts/Current Contents	**1990** Bioethicsline Drug Interactions UMLS GRATEFUL MED
1987 Drug/Poison Info Reconsider PDQ Internet Access Electronic News **1988** DXplain	**1991** Clinical Alerts NIH Guide E-mail **1992** Genetics Database Medical Facts File Faculty Publications

Databases at the Cutting Edge

Several medical libraries (and other types) have been in the forefront of library automation and share the limelight with Georgetown in pioneering efforts to develop and implement databases that represent the extended online catalog. This chapter is not intended, however, to review the literature. It is designed to present some of the Georgetown experience in providing databases at the cutting edge in order to provide the reader with ideas for databases to implement or to share.

Georgetown has followed several paths in database development and implementation. Some databases are developed entirely by Georgetown staff; some are ported in from other developers and loaded "as is"; and some are a combination of both. In addition, a few databases on the Knowledge Network reside on computers external to the Medical Library and to Georgetown University. In these instances, access is provided transparently to the user.

Databases Developed at Georgetown

All LIS databases, including the Online Catalog, miniMEDLINE, ALERTS™/Current Contents®, and Bioethicsline, have been developed at Georgetown. Multiple programming routines to sort, index, search, display, print, and download references and abstracts, as well as screen designs and searching capabilities have been developed, tested, and implemented by a staff team of librarians and programmers. (Database tapes are purchased from producers and vendors.) The Faculty Publications Database and the Medical Facts File are additional examples of databases whose content, design, and implementation originated at Georgetown.

Databases Ported In. Examples of databases Georgetown ports in and loads directly on its various computers, without embellishments, include the Drug and Poison Information System, Reconsider, DXplain, Clinical Alerts, NIH Guide, GRATEFUL MED, and the multiple files and software programs that comprise the Molecular Biology Databases.

Database Developed in Combination. Implementation of the Drug Interactions database was a combined effort. Programming staff at Georgetown made modifications to the vendor's single-user, PC-based product for a multi-user environment.

Databases External to the Medical Library and to Georgetown. If a user selects a database not available in-house, the Knowledge Network guides the user invisibly through dial-up access and user identification code sequences to the selected file. Georgetown's main campus and law center libraries maintain separate, and different, online systems from the Medical Center Library and from each other. Browing access is provided to both these catalogs for Knowledge Network users. The Genetic Databases, OMIM and GDB, are external to Georgetown and are located on computers at the Johns Hopkins University Welch Medical Library, in Baltimore, Maryland.

As shown in Figure 1, there are twenty-two databases currently available for Georgetown Knowledge Network users. These are divided into five categories: Bibliographic, Information/Factual, Diagnostic, Research, and Communications. Brief descriptions in the following section provide an overview of the database content, searching features for the user, and selected technical details about programming, file development, and updating schedules.

Bibliographic Databases

The development of the Knowledge Network at Georgetown had its roots in the bibliographic databases of the LIS. The implementation of the Online Catalog and subsequent end-user bibliographic databases from 1981 forward, are examples of a system that has potential for continued growth and expansion. Eight databases currently available on Georgetown's Knowledge Network are described in the following section.

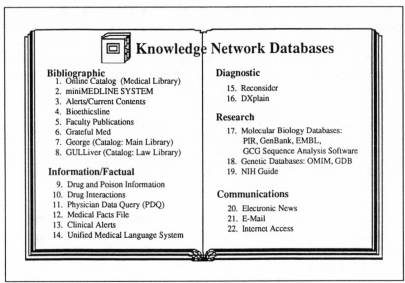

Figure 1. The single-menu access point to the libraries' Knowledge Network databases.

Online Catalog

At Georgetown, the Medical Center Library's Online Catalog with public access has been available since the fall of 1981 and provides the bibliographic records of all the print and non-print collections in the Library. The original design of this LIS component incorporated unique capabilities for keyword searching, in addition to subject searching using the Medical Subject Headings® (MeSH) as the subject authority. The design of the Online Catalog offers easy prompts for the user to search, display, and print references to the book, serial, audiovisual, and microcomputer software collections in the Medical Center Library.[31] Two added features of Georgetown's Online Catalog include the ability to browse the MeSH vocabulary file and the newly released Document Delivery System (DDS).

The advantage of browsing the MeSH file, as a menu option of the Online Catalog, gives users the ability to select subject headings, review online notes of a term's history and scope, and explode the categorized lists for context within a broader or narrower subject. Researchers often use this resource to provide MeSH terms and tree numbers for National Institutes of Health (NIH) grant applications. Reference staff teach health professionals the advantage of using the MeSH file to become familiar with the subject terminology in their specialty areas. This has proven to be important, particularly for users of the GRATEFUL MED software.

The newest feature of Georgetown's LIS is the DDS, introduced in 1991. It is designed with several entry points within LIS and can be accessed from the Online Catalog as well as other bibliographic databases. The DDS is totally electronic with predefined templates for a user to request books, book chapters, journal articles, and non-print resources. Each request is directed to the photocopy service or interlibrary loan service, depending on availability. If a user selects the DDS from the Online Catalog component and the item requested is not owned by the Library, then the template is filled out by the user. If access is made from any of the other bibliographic databases, such as miniMEDLINE or ALERTS/Current Contents, the template is automatically filled out by the system. In addition to requesting items, the DDS allows users to view the status of their pending requests and recommend purchases for the Library. Choices for delivery modes include pickup, mail, or fax; payment methods are selected by the requester to accommodate interdepartmental charges or cash transactions.

miniMEDLINE SYSTEM

The miniMEDLINE SYSTEM was introduced to the students, faculty, and staff at Georgetown in the summer of 1982 as one of the first self-service databases for users to conduct their own searches of the current biomedical literature. The concept focused on providing a resource for end-user searching, based on an in-house collection. The first miniMEDLINE file contained references from 120 key English language journals with emphasis in clinical specialties and covered the latest three years of the literature.[32]

The database is menu-driven and allows users to create search sets by author, title words, journal title, and MeSH subject terms. Once sets are created, a user manipulates the sets to refine the search strategy further, using Boolean OR and AND logic. The output from final search sets can be displayed on the screen, printed to paper, and downloaded to disc.

In 1982, MEDLINE tapes were not available from NLM, and the database content was derived from downloading references from monthly MEDLINE searches. Over the next few years, the miniMEDLINE journal coverage increased to 163 titles and broadened the subject scope in dentistry, nursing, and the basic sciences. In 1985, when the NLM released the MEDLINE tapes on a fee basis, Georgetown enhanced the miniMEDLINE software to extract references from the tapes and added abstracts.

The miniMEDLINE database has continued to grow during the ten years since its introduction, with more journal titles and years of coverage. Today, miniMEDLINE provides references and abstracts to articles from 1,164 journals, spans six years of coverage from April 1986 to the present, and contains close to 1.1 million references. Its extreme popularity and high use are evident in the number of searches conducted by users. During the 1982–83 academic year, use of the miniMEDLINE database totalled 11,234 search sessions. In 1991–92, over 33,000 searches were conducted.

ALERTS/Current Contents

In 1986, Georgetown introduced another end-user database into the Knowledge Network, ALERTS/Current Contents. Tapes were acquired from the Institute for Scientific Information in Philadelphia for two editions of Current Contents: Clinical Medicine and Life Sciences. Since Georgetown users of the Knowledge Network were familiar wih the searching menu and mechanics of miniMEDLINE, a similar approach was developed for this database. Software modifications were made, however, to suit the unique features of Current Contents. These features incorporated the ability to scan article titles from a specific journal issue, store a search profile, and use multiterm searching in one search statement with implied Boolean AND logic. The database is updated weekly and a one-year file is available.

The difference between the two databases, miniMEDLINE and ALERTS/Current Contents, is in journal coverage. The miniMEDLINE file is based on an in-house journal collection; ALERTS/Current Contents offers a combination of journal titles available in-house and others not in the Library collection. In ALERTS/Current Contents, each reference displayed indicates which journals the Library owns. For titles not in the Library, users have two choices: (1) they can request an interlibrary loan through the DDS; or (2) they can display the address for the senior author and request a reprint.

In 1988, the ALERTS/Current Contents database was increased from two to five editions. Subject coverage was expanded beyond clinical medicine and life sciences, into other topics including agriculture, biology, environment, physical, chemical, and earth sciences as well as engineering and technology disciplines. ALERTS/Current Contents currently covers 4,615 journal issues and has close to 59,000 references. Use of this database continues to grow, and it has been interesting to note that information seekers in the clinical specialties have been the most frequent users.

Bioethicsline

Bibliographers from the Kennedy Institute for Bioethics at Georgetown University, with funding from the NLM, compile the Bioethicsline database. In 1990, the Medical Center Library acquired the tapes from NLM and made the database available to Knowledge Network users. Bioethicsline uses similar menu, searching, and display features as miniMEDLINE and ALERTS/Current Contents, but it also provides additional notations for formats other than journal articles.

The file incorporates a wide variety of media and literary forms, including journal and newspaper articles, monographs, analytics, court decisions, bills, laws, and audiovisuals. Materials are selected from the literature of medicine, nursing, the biological sciences, philosophy, religion, law, and the behavioral sciences, as well as from the popular media. The database is comprehensive for English-language materials published from 1973 to the present and currently contains 32,911 citations.

Faculty Publications

Faculty Publications is a compilation of the scholarly achievements of the Georgetown University Medical Center faculty and academic staff. The Library has been compiling this annual publication since 1975 in a print format. In 1992, an online version was made available to Knowledge Network users.

The Faculty Publications Online provides references to the print and non-print publications by Georgetown University Medical Center faculty. Print publications include journal articles, books, book chapters, editorials, letters, and abstracts; non-print materials include microcomputer software and audiovisual programs. The file currently contains 2,500 listings for the 1990–91 academic year and can be searched by six categories: (1) Organization (e.g., School of Medicine, School of Nursing, Administration); (2) Department (e.g., Microbiology, Ophthalmology); (3) Author; (4) Publication Title (e.g., *New England Journal of Medicine*, *Principles of Internal Medicine*); (5) Title Words; and (6) Citation Type (e.g., book, journal article, editorial).

GRATEFUL MED

The GRATEFUL MED software is a front-end program designed to simplify the process of searching the NLM's MEDLINE database. In 1990, Georgetown acquired multiple copies of the GRATEFUL MED software and loaded them on an IBM 386 platform. This platform has the capability to run multiple virtual DOS or PC sessions and uses the Unix System V, release 3 software with DOS emulators.

Users can acess the GRATEFUL MED software through the Knowledge Network, but must have their own ID codes and passwords to use the NLM databases. Making the GRATEFUL MED software available on the Knowledge Network allows Georgetown users the capability for shared modem access and eliminates the need for a dedicated modem by individual users.

George (Main Library Catalog) and GULLiver (Law Library Catalog)

Each of the three campuses of Georgetown University—main, medical, and law—maintains a separate and independent library. Each library has its own, and different, online system. In 1990, the Medical Library offered Knowledge Network users access to the online catalogs of the main campus and law center libraries. The main campus library is on a contiguous campus to the Medical Library, and access to their online catalog, George, is available through the campus-wide AT&T ISN network. The Law Library is located seven miles from the Medical Library and access to their catalog, GULLiver, is accomplished through modem dial-up with connections made transparently for the user. Once access is made to each catalog, users are prompted by the online instructions unqiue for each system. To date, access from the other two online catalogs to the Medical Library catalog has not been implemented.

Informational/Factual Databases

Since the mid-1980s, Georgetown has continued to bring specialized information resources to its Knowledge Network users, particularly access to full-text information. Among the early examples are the Drug and Poison Information System, the Reconsider Diagnostic System, and the PDQ database of Cancer Treatment Information, all of which were implemented in 1987. In the following section, descriptions of six databases focus on a broadened scope for the Knowledge Network that goes beyond bibliographic into informational/factual databases.

Drug and Poison Information

Georgetown implemented the Drug and Posion Information database in 1987 and was one of the first libraries in the country to offer a multi-user version. Micromedex, Inc., the developers of the database, ported the system from a PC-based platform to the multi-user VAX environment for Georgetown. The database is updated quarterly. Screen displays and user commands for accessing the file are different from other Knowledge Network databases; however, users are guided by the system and have little difficulty in finding the latest drug and toxicology information.

This database has five separate files:

1. The Toxicology Information section contains ingredient information on over 750,000 commercial, industrial, pharmaceutical, and botanical substances. It provides over 800 detailed protocols to manage and treat reactions to ingested, dermal absorption, eye exposure, or inhalation of any of the listed substances.

2. The Drug Information portion provides detailed monographs for over 1,100 drugs and includes drug evaluations, adverse drug reactions, over 5,500 drug consults containing patient data and

clinical responses to different doses, and the Martindale Extra Pharmacopoeia for world-wide coverage of drugs in clinical use.

3. In the Disease and Trauma Information for Acute Care, data for the practice of acute care medicine is given, augmented with a 40,000 keyword medical thesaurus.

4. Aftercare Instructions offer suggestions to healthcare professionals on post-visit and post-treatment care with instructions in English and Spanish.

5. In the Reproductive Risk Information System, acute and chronic clinical, carcinogenic, genetic, and reproductive effects of chemicals and physical agents are provided.

Drug Interactions

The Drug Interactions database is derived from the Drug Therapy Screening System™ (DTSS), marketed by MEDI-SPAN, Inc. It is an interactive system that provides information of clinical significance on drug-drug interactions, food-drug interactions, and adverse drug reactions. The system also provides descriptive information about each drug. Three knowledge bases are available:

1. Mediphor provides drug-drug interactions, with data based on clinical evaluation of published reports on drug interactions.

2. Food-Drug, is similar to Mediphor, but provides appropriate warnings for established food-drug interactions of clinical significance.

3. PAR (Prior Adverse Reactions) documents previous adverse drug reactions and appropriate warnings to prevent recurrence in subsequent therapy.

Georgetown introduced the Drug Interactions database in 1990, as a complement to the Drug and Poison Information Sytem. The vendor's PC-based single-user system was modified by Georgetown programming staff to run in the multi-user environment of the Knowledge Network. The software is written in C. The file is updated quarterly.

Physician Data Query (PDQ)

In 1987, Georgetown became one of the first sites to implement the MUMPS version of PDQ and make it available to users of the Knowledge Network. The file is updated monthly and provides the most up-to-date information on clinically-oriented cancer information.

PDQ provides state-of-the-art cancer treatment information, descriptions of clinical trials, and directories of physicians and organizations providing cancer care. The database represents an effort by the National Cancer Institute to make known the latest cancer treatment information, facilitate access to clinical trials, and accelerate the practical application of advances in cancer research. The system is menu-driven and is divided into sections: (1) Cancer Information, (2) Directory, and (3) Protocols. The Protocol section contains summaries of more than 1,300 clinical trials currently accruing patients (active protocols), and more than thirty standard therapy protocols for the treatment of various types of cancer.

Medical Facts File

A newly developed database, the Medical Facts File, has been designed by Georgetown as an online source for users seeking quick answers to medical queries.[33] The concept for the database emerged from the Library's experience with commonly asked reference questions. Because information is widely scattered and users are faced with barriers of time and access, Georgetown is developing this database to give users a knowledge base of answers to common information queries asked in the library. The file is particularly useful during times when reference librarians are not available such as evenings and weekends, and for users accessing the Knowledge Network from remote sites. Plans are to introduce this database to Knowledge Network users in the fall of 1992.

The Medical Facts File anticipates questions by providing factual information and authoritative sources. The database is modular in design and is divided into eight sections:

1. Bioethics contains codes, oaths, and statements of ethical principles.
2. Diseases have descriptive summaries, eponyms, and schedules for immunizations, incubations, and isolations.
3. Directories includes the names and addresses of medical facilities and organizations.
4. History provides information on important medical discoveries, Nobel Prizes, and history of the Georgetown University Medical Center.
5. Publishing gives information on journals including instructions to authors, copyright, style manuals, and sample articles.
6. Statistics includes vital statistics, lab values, conversions, and weights and measures.
7. Terminology has abbreviations, acronyms, etymology, and prefixes/suffixes.

8. Scholarships contains summaries of approximately one hundred scholarships available to medical students.

The Publishing Module is the most fully developed portion of the file, to date, and currently contains information on fifty major journals of interest to the Georgetown faculty who publish. For each journal title, the information provided includes the title abbreviation, the sponsoring organization, editorial boards, peer review boards, copyright information, and instructions to authors. This information can be displayed, printed, or downloaded at a user's workstation. The Disease module is being developed and features summaries for the most often seen medical diagnosis at the Georgetown University Hospital, Division of Internal Medicine.

Within each of the eight modules, a number of subtopics are available and the user selects the specific topic by progressing through the hierarchical levels. A knowledgeable user, however, can go directly to a particular section by a subject approach. The database is being indexed with the UMLS Metathesaurus and provides an ideal platform for Georgetown to test the use of the UMLS as an intelligent retrieval tool for Knowledge Network users.

The Medical Facts File is programmed using SYBASE, a commercially developed database management software package. It runs on a Sun SPARC 490. The software was chosen to implement a combined menu and multiple window approach for user access that emphasizes easy user interface and intuitive searching mechanisms. Ease of use and transparent navigation is optimum because the system's goal is to provide self-service access to information and minimize the need for special training.

Clinical Alerts

Clinical Alerts provides electronic delivery of the results of NIH clinical trials prior to the published release in print format. The intent is to expedite dissemination of the information to health professionals. The online version of Clinical Alerts has been available for Georgetown users since 1991, with updates disseminated at irregular intervals.

Georgetown receives the Clinical Alerts by e-mail through the LISTSERVE distribution from the University of Maryland at Baltimore. Two types of dissemination are available. Georgetown users can access the file as a menu option on the Knowledge Network or they can arrange for facsimile transmission. The programming staff maintains the Clinical Alerts on an AT&T 3B2/500 platform. When a Clinical Alert is ready to be transmitted via fax, the text and a list of facsimile numbers are moved to a PC, equipped with an AT&T fax card. The Clinical Alert is then transmitted to appropriate fax numbers stored in the system. To date, there are forty-two Georgetown departments subscribing to this service.

Unified Medical Language System (UMLS)

Since 1990, Georgetown has offered Knowledge Network users an option for browsing the UMLS Metathesaurus. The version available is Meta-1 and contains all terms from the following eight sources:

1. 1990 MeSH, the NLM's Medical Subject Headings;
2. DSM-IIIR, the American Psychiatric Association's, *Diagnostic and Statistical Manual of Mental Disorders*, 3rd edition, revised;
3. selected terms from the MeSH Supplementary Chemical Records;
4. ICD-9, the *Internal Classification of Diseases*, 9th edition, Clinical Modification;
5. SNOMED, the College of American Pathologists' *Systematized Nomenclature of Medicine;*
6. the 1989 CPT, the American Medical Associations' *Current Procedural Terminology*;
7. LCSH, the Library of Congress Subject Headings; and
8. a set of clinical terms frequently used at three COSTAR implementations.

Diagnostic Databases

Diagnostic databases present an added dimension to Georgetown's Knowledge Network by providing the type of resource needed to teach medical decision making and problem solving to health professions students. Two diagnostic databases, Reconsider and DXplain, are intended to serve as diagnostic prompting systems and provide suggestions and guidance to the clinican-in-training in making appropriate differential diagnoses. The Library maintains other diagnostic systems that are workstation-dependent; these are used in controlled teaching environments and have limited use. The implementation of the diagnostic databases in the multi-user environment provides access to other health professionals, such as residents and fellows, and makes these resources available at many patient care sites.

Reconsider

When Georgetown implemented Reconsider in 1987, it was the first experience in providing a full-text database on the Knowledge Network. Reconsider is an interactive diagnostic prompting program which uses simple information retrieval techniques to generate a list of possible diseases. The knowledge base consists of full-text descriptions of 3,262 diseases from *Cur-*

rent Medical Information & Terminology (CMIT), 5th ed., 1981, published by the American Medical Association.

Users enter patient findings and medical terms, either words or phrases, and the program searches for these terms and their synonyms using an internal thesaurus. Each term is assigned a "selectivity" to measure its frequency of occurrence in the entire text. A term used in many disease descriptions ("pain") has a lower selectivity weight; however, a term occurring in only one or a few disease descriptions ("koplik") is more selective, and therefore has a higher weight. For each term, Reconsider computes a selectivity, and then adds that weight to every disease in which the term occurs. Diseases suggested by more terms, particularly by terms with high selectivity weights, will receive the highest scores. The implicated diseases are listed in decreasing order of total score. After generating a specific disease listing, the user can review the online text of the disease description from CMIT.

Even though the Reconsider database derives its information base from a 1981 textbook and does not have newer diseases, such as AIDS, faculty at Georgetown have found Reconsider to be helpful, in teaching the diagnosis of parasitic diseases, for which signs and symptoms have not changed that much since 1981. The patient population at the Georgetown University Hospital has an international profile because of the diplomatic, congressional, and other busineess groups that live, visit, and travel in and out of Washington, D.C. Reconsider is considered an important teaching tool to assist students in developing differential diagnosis skills for parasitic diseases.

DXplain

The second diagnostic system, DXplain, was introduced to Georgetown students in 1988 as a remote access database, available on computers at the Massachusetts General Hospital in Boston. Dial-up procedures and access codes were handled by the Knowledge Network software and long distance charges were absorbed by the Library. In Fall 1991, the database was brought to Georgetown and made available as an in-house file. Currently, it runs on an AT&T 386 platform and can accommodate eight simultaneous users.

DXplain provides access to a large database of signs and symptoms of different diagnoses, and reminds the user of disorders which might, in part, explain a set of clinical features entered by the user. DXplain includes a large number of common diseases as well as some rare diseases, for a combined total of over 2,000 diseases.

Research Databases

In 1989, Georgetown reached well beyond the bibliographic and information/ factual database level and began to offer a set of specialized databases to bench scientists engaged in genetic research. The same basic rules were applied to the selection of these databases. Ones with the highest potential for use were implemented, either as in-house systems or as dial-up databases with access gateways. The following three systems are examples of the Research Databases Georgetown now offers its users: Molecular Biology Databases, Genetic Databases, and the NIH Guide.

Molecular Biology Databases

Georgetown enlarged the scope of the Knowledge Network considerably in 1989, when it introduced the Molecular Biology Databases to its users. The group of databases, under the umbrella of Molecular Biology, includes a variety of sequence databases and sequence analysis software packages needed to search, manipulate, and match new sequences to published ones.

Currently, the following eight sequence database are available:

1. GenBank (Genetic Sequence Databank) contains more than 27,000 citations to journal articles and technical reports in genetic reseach, descriptions of DNA and RNA sequences with fifty or more nucleotide bases, and more 22,000 reported sequences totalling more than 26 million bases;

2. EMBL (European Molecular Biology Laboratory) Nucleotide Sequence Database contains about 44,000 nucleotide sequences covering approximately 56 million bases derived from eukaryote, prokaryote, virus, bacteriophage genetic DNA or RNA, MRNA, and functional RNA molecules;

3. NBRF-PIR (National Biomedical Research Foundation-Protein Identification Resource) Nucleic Acid Sequence Database with descriptions of approximately 4,000 genetic sequences in approximately 8 million bases including nucleic acid sequences for proteins and some regulatory and promoter sequences;

4. NBRF-PIR Protein Sequence Database with descriptions of more than 26,700 partial and whole protein sequences representing more than 7.6 million amino acids isolated or inferred from the gene sequences;

5. SWISS-PROT Protein Sequence Database contains descriptions of more than 10,000 nucleic acid and protein sequences;

6. VectorBank contains the nucleic acid sequences of 150 frequently used cloning vectors and restriction maps;

7. PROSITE, a dictionary of short motifs from protein sequences; and

8. REBASE, a file of restriction endonucleases and their restriction sites.

In addition to the sequence databases, Georgetown has acquired version 7.0 of the Genetics Computer Group (GCG) Sequence Analysis Software, the Kanehisa Homology Programs, and the NBRF Protein Sequence Query Software. All the sequence databases and sequence analysis software are maintained on the Library's VAX computers and researchers must make a special application to become subscribers. They must be Georgetown-based and on the Library's patron file, to qualify for space on the VAX. To date, over 130 scientists, including faculty, students, and staff in basic science and clinical specialties, are subscribers to the Molecular Biology databases. A centralized Hewlitt-Packard color plotter is available in the Library for users who do not have sequence plotting equipment. As a further help to users of the Molecular Biology databases, the Library sponsored a three-day workshop in May 1991, taught by the developers of the GCG Sequence Analysis Software. Fifty researchers and library staff registered for the workshop, held in the Library's computer classroom, and attended morning sessions of lectures and afternoon sessions that involved hands-on exercises.

Genetics Database

The two component files of the Genetics Database reside in computers at Johns Hopkins University and are examples of systems Georgetown provides for its Knowledge Network users through dial-up access. These are the latest research databases to became available and were implemented in 1992.

Genome Data Base (GDB) contains human gene mapping information. It is designed to collect, organize, store, and distribute data generated by scientists and has been implemented in the SYBASE relational database management system.

Online Mendelian Inheritance in Man (OMIM) is a full-text database of Dr. Victor A. McKusick's, *Mendelian Inheritance in Man*, and contains data on genetic disorders and traits.

NIH Guide

The NIH Guide is an invaluable resource to researchers who seek funding support for projects. The NIH Guide announces scientific initiatives and provides policy and administrative information to individuals and organizations who need to be kept informed of opportunities, requirements, and changes in extramural programs administered by the NIH.

In 1991, the Library became the dissemination point for the electronic version of the NIH Guide. It comes in a pre-formatted text file through e-mail, on a weekly basis. Programming staff at Georgetown parse the text file to modify the user display and print functions. The most recent four issues are kept online.

Communications Databases

As Georgetown increased the number and complexity of the databases offered on the Knowledge Network, it became essential to communicate electronically with users. A key factor in the communications process is the ability to transmit and receive news, mail, and other databases. The LIS Electronic News was introduced first, followed by the e-mail component, and finally, the Internet access which is currently under development and testing.

Electronic News. This provides a mechanism for the Library to make general announcements to users of the Knowledge Network concerning hours, resources, services, and special downtimes when database or computer maintenence is scheduled. It is used also by the Medical Center departments to announce items of broad interest such as grand rounds, special presentations by visiting faculty, and other university events. The Electronic News has been available since 1987 and announcements are handled by the Library's reference staff.

Electronic Mail. In 1991, Georgetown introduced an e-mail system to Knowledge Network users. E-mail uses a public domain package, ELM, modified by programming staff to suit the Georgetown environment.

Key features of the e-mail system at Georgetown include: (1) directory look-up of library patrons from the LIS Patron File; (2) the ability to send e-mail messages to colleagues on the Internet and BITNET; and (3) the ability to upload and download mail messages to and from a user workstation.

Internet Access. This component provides library patrons with a means to access Telnet and file transfer protocol (FTP) with other computers on the worldwide Internet network.

References

1. James Boswell, *Boswell's Life of Dr. Johnson,* Volume I (Oxford: Clarendon Press, 1887), 558.
2. P. B. Culkin, "Rethinking OPACS: the design of assertive information systems," *Information Technology and Libraries* 8 (June 1989): 172–77.
3. C. R. Hildreth, "Beyond boolean: designing the next generation of online catalogs," *Library Trends* 35 (Spring 1987): 647–67.
4. C. W. Bailey, "Public access computer systems: the next generation of library automation systems," *Information Technology and Libraries* 8 (June 1989): 178–85.
5. J. Drabenstott, J. Becker, G. K. Hartsough, W. Stahl, et al., "Beyond the online catalog: great potential and profound change," *Library Hi Tech* 6 (1988): 101–11.

6. P. Molholt, "Libraries and the new technologies: courting the Cheshire Cat," *Library Journal* 113 (November 15, 1988): 37–41.

7. E. Gallup-Fayen, "Microcomputers and the online catalog: changing how the catalog is used," *Journal of Educational Media and Library Sciences* 24 (Spring 1987): 230–41.

8. L. Jaffe, "The future of the online catalog: who decides?" *Online* 15 (January 1991): 7–9.

9. W. G. Potter, "Expanding the online catalog," *Information Technology and Libraries* 8 (June 1989): 99–104.

10. D. Avriel, R. Miller, and C. Ruchs, "The Israeli National Medical Library's new minicomputerized on-line integrated system (MAIMON)," *Bulletin of the Medical Library Association* 69 (April 1981): 216–23.

11. E. A. Kelly, D. K. Yedlin, S. Y. Crawford, and S. Igielnik, "On-line integrated library system: bibliographic access and control system of Washington University School of Medicine," *Bulletin of the Medical Library Association* 70 (July 1982): 281–88.

12. C. M. Goldstein, "Integrated library systems," *Bulletin of the Medical Library Association* 71 (July 1983): 308–11.

13. S. Y. Crawford, M. F. Johnson, and E. A. Kelly, "Technology at Washington University School of Medicine library: BACS, PHILSOM, and OCTANET," *Bulletin of the Medical Library Association* 73 (July 1983): 324–27.

14. N. C. Broering, "The Georgetown University Library Information System (LIS): a minicomputer-based integrated library system," *Bulletin of the Medical Library Association* 71 (July 1983): 317–23.

15. D. Avriel, "The library and its home computer: automation as if people mattered," *Bulletin of the Medical Library Association* 71 (July 1983): 328–37.

16. N. C. Broering, "Introduction: high technology in health sciences libraries," *Bulletin of the Medical Library Association* 71 (July 1983): 306–7.

17. C. L. Jones and D. B. Marcum, "Integrated systems: from library to campus and beyond," *Bulletin of the Medical Library Association* 71 (July 1983): 338–42.

18. E. A. Kelly, B. Halbrook, S. Igielnik, and C. Rueby, "BACS: evolution of an integrated library system toward information management," *Bulletin of the Medical Library Association* 73 (January 1985): 9–14.

19. S. Y. Crawford, B. Halbrok, E. A. Kelly, and L. Stucki, "Beyond the online catalog: developing an academic information system in the sciences," *Bulletin of the Medical Library Association* 75 (July 1987): 202–8.

20. Crawford, "Beyond the online catalog," 202–8.

21. N. C. Broering, "The miniMEDLINE SYSTEM: a library-based end-user search system," *Bulletin of the Medical Library Association* 73 (April 1985): 138–45.

22. N. C. Broering and B. Cannard, "Building bridges: LIS-IAIMS-BioSYNTHESIS," *Special Libraries* 79 (Fall 1988): 302–13.

23. G. M. Pitkin, "Access to articles through the online catalog," *American Libraries* 19 (October 1988): 769–70.

24. F. Wilson, "Article-level access to the online catalog at Vanderbilt University," *Information Technology and Libraries* 8 (June 1989): 121–31.

25. G. S. Machovec, "Locally loaded databases in Arizona State University's online catalog using the CARL system," *Information Technology and Libraries* 8 (June 1989): 161–71.

26. Unified Medical Language System™, National Library of Medicine Fact Sheet. November 1991. 2 pages.

27. N. C. Broering, H. R. Gault, and H. Epstein, "BioSYNTHESIS: bridging the information gap," *Bulletin of the Medical Library Association* 77 (January 1989): 19–25.

28. N. C. Broering, H. E. Bagdoyan, J. S. Hylton, and J. Rosansky, "A demonstration of BioSYNTHESIS, a system integration tool for multiple databases." *Proceedings of the Fourteenth Annual Symposium on Computer Applications in Medical Care*, Washington D.C., November 4–7, 1990 (New York: IEEE, 1990), 961–64.

29. N. C. Broering, J. S. Hylton, R. Guttmann, and D. Eskridge, "BioSYNTHESIS: access to a knowledge network of health sciences databases," *Journal of Medical Systems* 15 (April 1991): 139–53.

30. Broering, "The miniMEDLINE SYSTEM," 138–45.

31. Broering, "The Georgetown University Library Information System," 317–23.

32. Broering, "The miniMEDLINE SYSTEM," 138–45.

33. N. C. Broering, H. E. Bagdoyan, D. Fagan, J. S. Hylton, and R. Guttmann, "Medical Facts File: a self-service database of reference information." *Proceedings of the Fifteenth Annual Symposium on Computer Applications in Medical Care*, Washington D.C. November 7–20, 1991 (New York: McGraw-Hill, Inc. 1992), 886–88.

Chapter 10.
Managing Information in Biomedical
Research: The Human Genome Project

Susan Crawford
*Professor of Biomedical Communication and
Director, Library and Biomedical Communications Center
Washington University School of Medicine*

Loretta Stucki
*Associate Director, Technical Services
and Network Administration
Library and Biomedical Communications Center
Washington University School of Medicine*

Barbara Halbrook
*Deputy Director
Library and Biomedical Communications Center
Washington University School of Medicine*

Abstract

*With the dominance of molecular biology in biomedical research, genetic data-
bases are among the most important in the biological sciences. Genetic research,
both basic and clinical, cuts across many specialties and vast amounts of information must be accessed and managed. The National Center for Biotechnology
Information (NCBI) is responsible for coordinating and standardizing genome
sequencing information on a global basis. One of seven organizations designated
by the National Institutes of Health as a research center for the National Human
Genome Project, Washington University serves as a test site for the NCBI database. The library manages access for the university's biomedical scientists and
provides organized feedback to NCBI on the operation of the databases.*

*At their 1991 annual meeting in London, 700 scientists in genome re-
search reported abstracts of their work in a volume that numbered over 350
pages. The effort to map the human genome clearly shows how biomedical*

research is being conducted in the era of big science and how difficult are the problems in handling massive amounts of data.

Background

The international effort in mapping the human genome originated from biological advances that accelerated during the mid-1980s. As reported by Watson, former director of the Human Genome Project, the Department of Energy (DOE) was concerned, at that time, with the problem of detecting inherited mutations resulting from the use of atomic bombs in Hiroshima and Nagasaki.[1] An influential article in *Science* suggested that sequencing the human genome would be an excellent way to expedite cancer research.[2] It has been estimated that some 4,000 diseases have genetic components, ranging from Alzheimer's disease to childhood cancer.[3] The notion of a systematic approach to identifying all human genes was endorsed both by DOE in 1987 and by the National Research Council in 1988, with recommendations for a $200 million annual budget over several years.[4] The international scientific community quickly responded by developing genome programs in France, Italy, the United Kingdom, and the former U.S.S.R. In the United States, Congress began funding the Human Genome Project in 1988. With annual increases, appropriations to the National Institutes of Health (NIH) were estimated to reach $87.5 million by 1991 and appropriations to DOE would reach $47.7 million.[5] In 1990, an international scientific organization, the Human Genome Organization (HUGO) was formed.

As of May 1991, seven institutions had been designated by NIH as centers of investigation for the federally funded human genome initiative: Baylor College of Medicine, Children's Hospital of Philadelphia, Massachusetts Institute of Technology, University of California at San Francisco, University of Michigan, University of Utah, and Washington University. Each center is assigned to work on one or several chromosomes and acts as a resource for scientists working at other laboratories. While these centers have been charged with deciphering the complete genetic message of humans at the molecular level, there are many laboratories and clinical departments that are working on other aspects. Projects include mapping the location of genes responsible for specific diseases and conditions such as cystic fibrosis and Down's syndrome. Other studies attempt to correlate genetic and environmental factors, as in alcoholism and schizophrenia.

Flow of Information and Creation of Databases

The major product of the Human Genome Project is a series of linked data sets containing the genetic and physical location of all genes on each chromosome, and the complete nucleotide sequence of the genome for humans and several model organisms, as outlined by Pearson and Söll:[6]

- constructing a high-resolution genetic map of the human genome;
- producing a variety of physical maps of all human chromosomes and the chromosomes of selected model organisms;
- determining the complete sequence of DNA in humans and in selected model organisms;
- developing capabilities for collecting, storing, distributing, and analyzing the data produced; and
- creating appropriate technologies necessary to achieve these objectives.

A formidable body of data that must be collected, analyzed, and distributed is being generated from the project. Journal publication is still important in communicating results and in staking a claim to findings, but changes in the communications system are emerging: the development of electronic databases and the transfer of information through telecommunications networks. As indicated in Figure 1, data are generated by scientists in electronic format and input into local databases. The data are then entered into specialized or global databases that are accessible to the scientific community.[7]

By content, the public access databases containing genome information may be divided into those dealing with maps, sequences, or bibliographic data.

Mapping information is compiled at Johns Hopkins University. Data from laboratories are received through Internet and Telenet and screened by a committee before entering into the Genome Data Base (GDB). The information is correlated with Online Mendelian Inheritance in Man (OMIM), a compendium of published information on human genetic diseases. When a scientist enters data into GDB, a sequential number is assigned, which establishes priority and at the same time indicates that the data has been validated. Increasingly, journals will not publish a paper unless there is a sequential number assigned to the data by GDB. As of November 1991, a CD-ROM version of GDB was considered.[8]

Sequence information is handled by global databases in the United States (NCBI—National Center for Biotechnology Information, National Library of Medicine), Europe (EMBL—European Molecular Biology Laboratory Data Library), and Japan (DDBJ—DNA Databank of Japan). They maintain all known DNA and RNA sequences from any organism and they have an international agreement to exchange information. Initially, only published sequences were handled, but the information banks now accept data. Presently, these databases contain more than 65 million sequenced DNA and RNA base pairs from 3,000 species, including complete genomes of some 200 organelles,

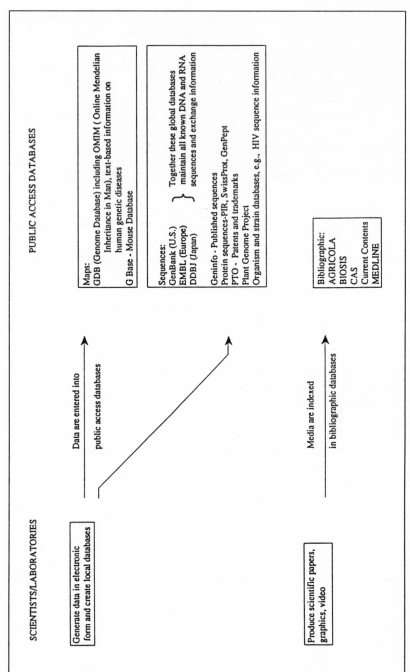

Figure 1. Flow of information and creation of databases in the Genome Project

viruses, and plasmids. In addition, there are specialized databases, among them, for protein sequences, for organism or strain, and for diseases such as HIV.

Bibliographic databases identify relevant papers published in scientific journals in agriculture, biology, chemistry, medicine, and the general sciences.

The National Library of Medicine Genetic Database

With the proliferation of databases, a major challenge is linkage of the three data sets so that information is readily accessible to the scientific community. This involves standardizing data representation and developing an infrastructure, transparent to the user, to retrieve and deliver needed information.

Beginning in 1992, NCBI, a branch of the U. S. National Library of Medicine (NLM), assumed responsibility for creating a unified database for sequences (see Figure 2). Data from Los Alamos, EMBL, DDBJ, MEDLINE, and direct submission by scientists is input into the NCBI database. The data is mapped into a standard international descriptor language called "abstract-syntax notation.1" (ASN.1). Developed by NCBI, ASN.1 is capable of expressing complicated biological relationships. NCBI plans to make its sequence database available through online access and CD-ROM. Called EN-TREZ, the CD-ROM system will be available through subscription with quarterly updates. Being developed also are ASN tools, a system of software for manipulating the database.

Through national and international communications networks such as Internet, scientists can access genome databases or deposit data directly from

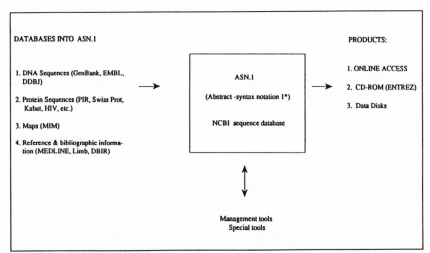

Figure 2. Genetics databases coordinated by the National Center for Biotechnology Information, National Library of Medicine, January 1992

their laboratories. The entire NCBI sequence database may be used online or purchased on CD-ROM disks and stored locally. Within medical centers, these and other databases are increasingly being downloaded into mini- or mainframe computers to be accessed by many users. Through the networks, updates of the data can now be made online, replacing the mailing of tapes and CD-ROMs.

Analysis of the data requires sophisticated mathematical and computational techniques. Software packages have been developed by several groups, among them, NCBI, Genetics Computer Group (GCG), Intelligenetics, and Beckman. Databases are searched for such relationships as correlations, anomalies, similarities, and co-occurrences. The ability to electronically explore databases is a powerful tool for discovery.[9]

Also shown in Figure 1, scientists access and use genome data prior to publication of that data. Information is peer reviewed by a committee before entering into public access databases. However, mapping information is presently accumulating so rapidly that intermediary unscreened databases, prior to entering into the Johns Hopkins Genome Database, have been suggested, in order to cut the time delay.[10] An additional problem is the complexity of electronic databases. While they present new and efficient approaches to data analysis, they require collaboration among scientists, computer specialists, statisticians, and others.

Making Genetic Databases Available at Washington University

The Washington University (WU) Medical Center supports a broad-based program in genetics research. The University is one of seven organizations designated by the NIH as a research center for the national Human Genome Project. Over 300 laboratories at the center are involved in some type of genetic research, ranging from large-scale collaborative efforts to scientists in small laboratories.

The Medical Library was approached by scientists to develop a program that would:

- provide the Medical Center access to databases that relate to genome sequencing and mapping, beginning with those that are most relevant to research at the Center;
- develop a communications infrastructure, transparent to the user, that will enable access to in-house, local, and remote databases, and to relevant telecommunications networks;
- mount locally and network these databases to departments within the Medical Center and provide selected software for data analysis; and
- provide training and staff support for use of the data.

In response to these needs, WU Medical Library entered into an agreement with NCBI to become a test site for its GenInfo online search system. GenInfo coordinates some twenty databases that contain mapping and sequencing information. It presently includes other databases on cloning vectors, macromolecular structures, molecular biology databases, and biotechnology information resources. GenInfo is part of an ongoing program for developing software tools to support research in genetics and molecular biology.

The agreement provides WU scientists free online access to the GenInfo database. WU will provide organized feedback to NCBI on user interface with the system and the software—its general usability, amount of assistance needed by the scientists, parts of the system that are problematic, and whether there are unmet needs. NCBI wishes to have data to project the load on its system before making it available nationwide. WU Medical Library will coordinate the program and act as liaison between NCBI and the users. The project coordinator will manage software packages, hardware requirements, and the Ethernet and Internet protocols that support access to GenInfo. The Library will also be responsible for passwords to GenInfo and for teaching use of the databases through workshops, seminars, individual instruction, and manuals.

Accessing GenInfo

Access to GenInfo is being developed in two phases at Washington University: direct online access and availability through the Bibliographic Access and Control System (BACS) (see Figure 3).

Direct online access by scientists is available through the Internet. Some fifty access codes are provided by NCBI to individual scientists who will access GenInfo from their laboratories or offices.

Direct online access is also available through the Library's BACS information system from a special workstation located in its Information Services area.

During a later phase of the project, selected genome databases or subsets from NCBI, as well as locally produced databases, will be loaded onto the Medical Center computers and made accessible through the BACS network. A customized menu will prompt selection from the total services and databases available through the BACS system.

GenInfo databases will be updated bimonthly by downloading data directly from NCBI to a local fileserver using ftp (file transfer protocol) via the Internet. Search software from NCBI will be used for the local installation at the Medical Center. Additional search software (e.g., Genetics Computer Group) will be leased or purchased to provide users with as many search options as possible. As the Internet, now operating at 10 megabits per second, is upgraded to 1 gigabit per second, the local database will be updated more

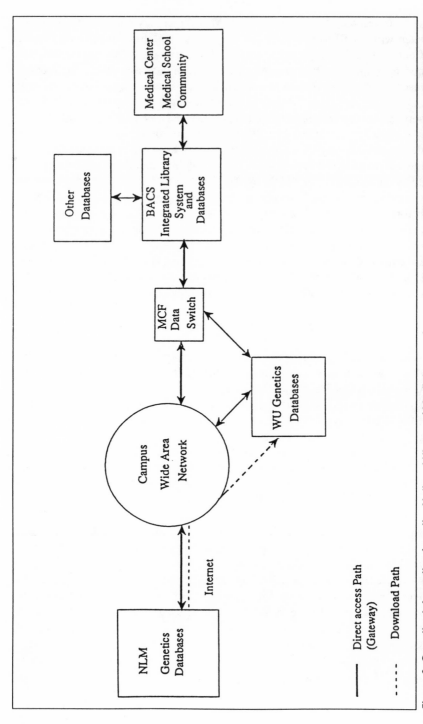

Figure 3. Genetics Information from the National Library of Medicine reaches users (1) through a direct access gateway or (2) through a locally maintained database at Washington University that is networked through the library's BACS system.

frequently. The high-speed network will also allow a graphically oriented approach to retrieving information from GenInfo.

The BACS system also connects with the campus-wide network to provide a gateway for other departments of WU that are not situated at the Medical Center.

Conclusion

With the dominance of molecular biology in biomedical research, genetic databases are among the most important in the biological sciences. Genetic research, both basic and clinical, cuts across many specialty areas. Vast amounts of information are being generated that must be accessed and managed before publication. In 1991, the NCBI assumed the responsibility for coordinating and standardizing genome sequencing information on a global basis.

While NCBI provides the infrastructure for handling genetic information, it is the role of other organizations to develop programs to meet the needs of specific research efforts. This chapter reports the role of the library as a point of focus and clearinghouse for genetic information in a large academic research center.

The WU Library and Biomedical Communications Center coordinates a program for providing access to both bibliographic and non-bibliographic databases. Genome data is accessed online and downloaded into its BACS-integrated information system, and networked throughout the Medical Center. The Library assumes responsibility for managing the database and for providing user support services. User training is an important aspect of the program, as is providing selected software for handling the data. The project serves as a model for new directions in library programming and for responding to research needs.

Dr. David Lipman, director of NCBI, agrees that the library is the appropriate administrative unit for coordinating the genome information program. He suggested that the library serves as the funnel for organized feedback from scientists to NCBI on database use and problems. The response of users is especially important for determining future development and the library plays an important role.

Plans include expansion of the database and its enhancement through software development, as needed by the scientists. The kinds of technological support required by the library and the need for special training of the staff will be explored. The program provides a base for investigating issues relating to information management in libraries as they are challenged with new roles.

References

1. J. D. Watson and R. M. Cook-Deegan, "Origins of the Human Genome Project," *FASEB Journal* 5 (January 1991): 8–9.
2. R. Dulbecco, "A turning point in cancer research: sequencing the human genome," *Science* 231 (March 7, 1986): 1055–56.
3. Genetics: Breaking life's code. 1990 Annual Report. Washington University Medical Center in St. Louis. Washington University (1991), 2.
4. Watson and Cook-Deegan, "Origins of the Human Genome Project," 9.
5. Watson and Cook-Deegan, "Origins of the Human Genome Project," 9–10.
6. M. L. Pearson and D. Söll, "The Human Genome Project: a paradigm for information management in the sciences," *FASEB Journal* 5 (January 1991): 35–36.
7. Pearson and Söll, "The Human Genome Project," 37–38.
8. Memorandum from Judy Adkinson, Johns Hopkins University Press, November 6, 1991.
9. E. Bradley and R. Tibshirani, "Statistical data analysis in the computer age," *Science* 253 (July 26, 1991): 390–95.
10. P. Aldhous, "Human genome databases at the crossroads," *Nature* 352 (July 11, 1991): 94.

CHAPTER 11.
THE OPAC AND IMAGE WORKSTATIONS

Wilma A. Bass
Coordinator of Cataloging Systems
Georgetown University Medical Center

Abstract

A possible component of the networked library of tomorrow will be the image workstation. X-rays, slides, or hard copy will be digitized and stored. These digitized images will be indexed, and catalog records will be linked to each image. Existing cataloging standards must be expanded and revised to adapt to this new media. New indexing terms must be established to specifically indicate the details of each image. As these expanded databases develop and become a standard resource, librarians will be encouraged to keep abreast of new technological advances in order to provide patrons with information quickly and efficiently.

Introduction

The progression from card catalogs to online public catalogs is now being extended to include digitized images. The complexity of name authority files, tag validation, and journal check-in has been conquered. Today, technology allows the librarian to face the challenge of developing image workstations which will provide indexed access to digitized image collections. At first glance, this new format of displaying information could seem overwhelming, but by retracing our steps and building on previous experiences, we can adapt and expand our knowledge and resources.

As early as 1934, Otlet wrote that "document" denotes not just books in the usual sense, but any expression of human thought. By 1951, Briet stated that bibliographic and information retrieval no longer dealt with texts but with access to evidence. These two concepts have advanced information technology to include image handling.[1] Today images can be handled in the same manner as other physical medium, such as sound and text. Access to information can now extend via the online catalog to include all images in digitized format.

Imaging offers unique features that other technologies do not possess:

1. It allows fast access to and retrieval of the document image.
2. It allows automated retrieval by linking a bibliographic search with an image database.
3. The digital image file can be compressed and compactly stored.
4. The digital image file may be restored although the original media may deteriorate given time.[2]

Digitized Image Workstations

Several factors must be taken into account to create digitized image workstations. The images should maintain a high quality of textual and graphic information. The cost of transferring the image should be economical. Images should be readily accessed and retrieved. Linkage between the item and descriptive information must occur.

A variety of alternative workstations are available for retrieving information including the terminal, full-function workstation, and local server models.

The Terminal Model

A dumb terminal with high-resolution graphics display is controlled directly by the host supporting the image database. The host sends pixels instead of characters.

The Full-Function Workstation Model

The user has a full-function workstation. Selected images are transferred as files from the image database host to the local workstation. Display and printing of the image are executed on the workstation without further interaction with the host. Actual copies of images can be stored on a long-term basis on the local workstation.

The Local Server Model

The central image database transmits remote directives and data across the network. The workstation performs a significant amount of local processing, but in continuous and close cooperation with the host supporting the central image database. Images are never formally transferred to the workstation or stored there. The central host transmits data that appears on the workstation screen via the display server software running in the workstation[3] (see Figure 1).

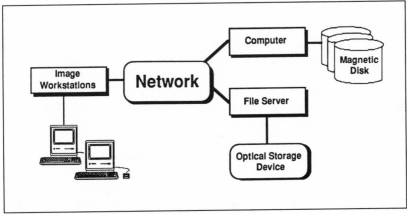

Figure 1. Local server workstation model

Creating an Image Database

The initial step in creating an image database is to assign a unique identifier to the hard copy when it is originally scanned. This unique identifier, similar to an LC card number, ISSN, or MARC number, will serve as the linkage between the image and its corresponding citation. The specific image (X-ray, picture, slide) can be digitized using a flat-bed scanner, photo-digitizing camera, slide scanner or video board (see Figure 2). Each image is scanned separately and the new digitized image is saved as an individual file. The file can be stored on hard disk, CD, tape, or cartridge. Due to the large amount of space required to store an image, they are grouped and generally stored on large-capacity hard

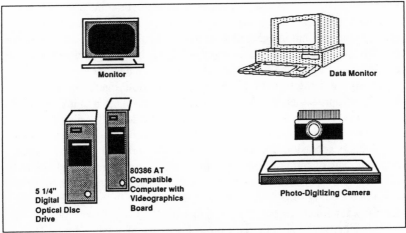

Figure 2. Imaging capture and display equipment

drives and accessed by the user at the workstation by one of the alternative models previously discussed.

The patron searching the database would enter specific search terms. Citations are retrieved and if an image is linked to the particular citation, the user is informed. The user selects specific citations, which will display an image along with the bibliographic information. The patron then has the option to print the complete citation, including the image. An image manipulation function allows the image displayed to be zoomed, reduced, rotated, or panned.

Examples of Image Databases

Library administrators recognized the value of having computer systems display images of items in their collections in the late 1980s. Access to these on-screen images allows users to recognize an image quickly. Being able to see the images will prevent the problem of retrieving the incorrect item. No catalog record, complete with textual description, can substitute for viewing an image of the item itself. Many museums, archives, and libraries have art collections which are either too large, too small, or too fragile both to attach cataloging information to them and retrieve them easily when someone requests them. The most important automation problem in these collections is their vast number of items. Cataloging and imaging such a collection is an immense task.[4]

The ArchiVISTA Project

The National Archives of Canada developed an optical disk imaging system which merged imaging technology with an existing database. Archi-VISTA, available to the public in June 1989, provided access to more than 20,000 editorial cartoons and caricatures in the archives collection. The system was built on the knowledge and experience of those involved in both bibliographic databases and imaging technology.

In April 1983, the archives began computerizing the catalog records of its collection. Begun in September 1988, the image capture system consisted of a photo-digitizing camera, an IBM AT compatible microcomputer with a VISTA videoprocessor board, VGA controller, an image monitor, a 14-inch data monitor, and Laserdrive 5 1/4-inch digital WORM optical disk drive. Each scanned image was stored in the videoprocessor's buffer and assigned essential control data: accession and item number of the original drawing, operator name, and date of capture. The accession and item number, uniquely identifying every holding within the collection, provides the necessary link to the corresponding catalog record and displayed this number in the upper right-hand corner of each image written to optical disk drive.

Originally, the ArchiVISTA project was planned using digital WORM optical disk for image retrieval, but the use of videodisc technology was proposed as as superior means of meeting or exceeding the specified speed and resolution for display and printing. The user interface, which provides a fully bilingual database, allows the user to browse or specify one or more of the following access points: subject, artist, publication, place, date, and unique item numbers. When a search is executed, the user is provided the option of modifying the search parameters or viewing the hit file of images and corresponding descriptive records. Display time will hopefully be reduced from seven seconds to three seconds. The user can also pan across or zoom in on a portion of a selected image using a mouse. The equivalent of newspaper quality images can be printed on ordinary bond paper using a standard laser printer specially equipped to reproduce one hundred lines per inch halftone images.[5]

The National Agricultural Library and forty-two land grant libraries have entered into a cooperative project to test a new method of capturing full text and images in digital format for publication on CD-ROM laser disks. The project will evaluate a turnkey scanning system to determine if it is now possible to provide in-depth access to the literature of agriculture while at the same time preserving it from rapid deterioration. The system utilizes a scanning methodology which coverts full text, including graphics and illustrations, to a bit-mapped digitized page image which then coverts the text to digitized ASCII code. The ASCII code is then processed by computer software and indexed. The resulting digitized text, bit-mapped page images, and indexes can be stored on a variety of electronic storage devices for retrieval on microcomputer workstations.

For purposes of this project, a "document" will consist of a book chapter, journal article, or other similar section of a whole piece. The document itself will consist of all of the text for that document including title, author, chapter number, and other applicable information. A full MARC catalog record will be available on the CD-ROM disks for each scanned publication. When the publication is a full book or journal, the standard cataloging records will be used. However, when an individual article or chapter is the only part of a larger work on the disk, then a MARC catalog record will be created for that article or chapter. Relational headers, the descriptive records necessary for system control and searching, identify a document within the system. They are input to the system as each document is scanned. Linkage occurs between the relational headers to both the associated documents and the MARC records. Linkages will allow the user to get directly to all other chapters in a book, after retrieving a specific chapter. Another link will connect a host item table of contents with each document allowing users to browse a table of contents and go directly to the chapter of interest. A final link will connect the ASCII version of a document to the bit-mapped page images, so that users can view associated images.[6]

Cataloging this new material, as well as making it accessible and retrievable is presently a challenge. Each new image entering the database reflects a variety of sources and subject areas, each with its own controlled vocabulary or specific requirements. Maps require coordinates; paintings, do not. In addition, image databases tend to contain local information, such as the name of a donor or how the image was obtained. There are no specific guidelines for cataloging image collections. Images existing in a digital format do not have a physical dimension, as do the slides they were scanned from. The physical description of a digitized item should include information containing the mode of scanning, resolution, file size, and file format. Some catalogers do use the MARC Audiovisual Materials format to catalog image collections, but many find this format inadequate[7] (see Figure 3).

Rensselaer Polytechnic's Architecture Library

At Rensselaer Polytechnic Institute's Architecture Library, catalogers discovered the need to standardize cataloging practices and descriptive terminology to improve consistency when they began a project of cataloging their entire collection of approximately 70,000 slides. Extensive cross-referencing was needed to improve retrieval time. The MARC-OCLC audiovisual media format was

Marc Tag and Subfield	Definition and Example
049 a GTUD	Holding Library
059 a 000013	Library Unique Identifier
096 a QZ 17 C576 No.3431 DI	Call Number
245 a h #a Dominant hemisphere language dysfunction #h [digitized image].	Title Statement Title Proper Media Designator
260 a b c #a Summit, N.J.: #b Ciba-Geigy, #C 1973.	Imprint Place of Production Name of Producer Year of Production
300 a b c d e #a 1 digitized image: #b PICT; #c 8-bit col., #d 72 DPI; 325k	Physical Description Extent of Item File Format Model of Scanning Resolution File Size
440 a v #a Ciba collection of medical illustrations; #v no. 3431	Series Statement Series Title Series Number
650 a x #a Aphasia #x CT scan	Subject Headings Topical Heading Form Qualifier

Figure 3. Digitized image MARC format

converted to make the slide database more compatible with Rensselaer's online information system. Redefining fields and subfields was required.[8]

Not every image will fit neatly into the criteria used by MARC to define its fields and subfields. Often, the cataloger is forced to reinterpret and expand the MARC field definitions in a very open-ended manner. At Rensselaer, in deciding to use MARC field codes and definitions, consistency and compatibility were gained; however, some flexibility and a measure of control over their own work process was sacrificed.

NASA-Johnson Space Center

The inherent problem of image retrieval within many visual collections is both the sparsity and inconsistency of subject assignment. The film repository at the NASA-Johnson Space Center (JSC) in Houston, Texas houses a collection of more than 1 million negatives and transparencies, as well as around 10,000 motion picture and audio reels, documenting all aspects of the U.S. manned space flight program since 1958. The JSC film repository discovered subject-access discrepancies due to the time span of its collection. Partly, this was attributed to the evolving vocabulary as programs within the agency matured, but primarily it was due to the highly subjective nature of describing image content. The viewpoint of the cataloger invariably changes from week to week and most often differs from the perspective of the engineer or the scientist. The wider the disparity in the points of view, the less likely the appropriate item will be retrieved.[9]

Georgetown University's Medical Center Library

At Georgetown University's Medical Center Library, the possibility of digitizing the slide collection of the Ciba Collection of Medical Illustrations was studied. Having previously experimented with formats that predated MARC standards, the cataloging staff was familiar with adapting existing tags and subfields for a model MARC-format. For example, a 300 tag providing a description of size in inches does not apply to an image measured in bits. The 300 field in this MARC format will be re-assigned as:

- Subfield b. The format for displaying images on a Macintosh computer (PICT or TIFF).
- Subfield c. Bit size and color, the mode of scanning and color information, that includes the number of colors, gray scale, or black and white (8-bit color).
- Subfield d. The image resolution in dots per inch (72dpi).
- Subfield e. File size (352k).

Even the media format designation had to change from "slides" to "digitized image."

The biggest challenge came in examining subject access for this new media. The National Library of Medicine's (NLM) Medical Subject Headings® (MeSH) and qualifiers are assigned to all items in the Medical Center Library's collection. The MeSH form qualifier "slides" was not an appropriate description of the new media. Furthermore, the existing topical qualifiers could not adequately reflect the detail of a digitized image or describe the technique used to create the parent image. For example, a user would need to know the type of stain used on tissue cells displayed in the image. By developing new qualifying terms such as schema, light photomicography, or gross anatomy, these techniques and concepts could be expressed in the catalog record (see Figure 4). Resources such as the Unified Medical Language System® (UMLS) may provide the sources for librarians to expand their knowledge of terms for use in indexing and lead to expanded controlled vocabularies.

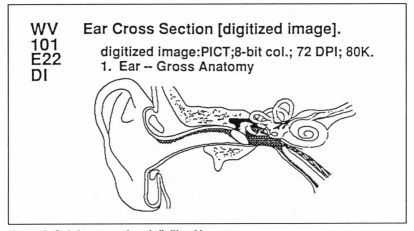

WV
101
E22
DI

Ear Cross Section [digitized image].

digitized image:PICT;8-bit col.; 72 DPI; 80K.
1. Ear -- Gross Anatomy

Figure 4. Catalog record and digitized image

At present, this project is in its initial stage of development, but once the material is scanned, storage and efficient retrieval facilitated, and cataloging completed, another valuable resource will be made accessible through the computer.

References

1. Michael K. Buckland, "Information retrieval of more than text," *Journal of the American Society for Information Science* 42 (8) (1991): 586–88.

2. George R. Thoma and Frank L. Walker, "Archiving the biomedical literature by electronic imaging methods," *ASIS '88: Information Technology: Planning for the Next 50 Years* (25) (1988): 132–36.
3. Clifford A. Lynch, "Image retrieval, display and reproduction," 9th National On-line Meeting, (May 1988): 227–32.
4. Howard Besser, "Imaging: fine arts," *Journal of the American Society for Information Science* 42(8) (1991): 589–96.
5. Gerald Stone and Philip Sylvain, "ArchiVISTA: a new horizon in providing access to visual records of the National Archives of Canada," *Library Trends* 38 (Spring 1990): 737–50.
6. Pamela Q. J. Andre and Nancy L. Eaton, "National agricultural text digitizing project," *Library Hi Tech* 6(3) (1988): 61–66.
7. Howard Besser, "Image databases," *Annual Review of OCLC Research* (June 1991): 49–50.
8. Jeanne M. Keefe, "The image as document: descriptive programs at Rensselaer," *Library Trends* 38 (Spring 1990): 659–81.
9. Gary A. Seloff, "Automated access to the NASA-JSC image archives," *Library Trends* 38 (Spring 1990): 682–96.

Chapter 12.
Partnering in the 1990s:
The Montefiore Medical Center and
The Albert Einstein College of Medicine
Collaborate on Library Automation

Josefina P. Lim
Library Director
Robert and Phyllis Tishman Learning Center
Montefiore Medical Center

James Swanton
System Manager
D. Samuel Gottesman Library
Albert Einstein College of Medicine

Abstract

The institutional backgrounds of the Montefiore Medical Center's (MMC) Tishman Learning Center (TLC) and the Albert Einstein College of Medicine's (AECOM) Gottesman Library are described and highlights of a consultant team's report, which led to an administrative agreement for shared information resources between the two institutions are discussed. The local area network connectivity specifications for the TLC are provided in detail. Also described is the decision making process for choosing the Georgetown University™ Library Information System as the MMC-AECOM multilibrary system of choice and the successful installation and implementation at the two libraries. Future plans include prospects for medical informatics at TLC.

Institutional Background

The Montefiore Medical Center (MMC) is a 1,256-bed primary health resource facility in the Bronx, New York. It is a major teaching affiliate of the Albert Einstein College of Medicine (AECOM), incorporating two acute-care hospitals, family health centers, home health services, nursing homes, a municipal hospital, and other facilities with approximately 10,000 staff and students. The MMC Library subscribes to 851 current serial titles and has a monographic collection of 15,000 volumes and an internationally renowned archives collection.

The D. Samuel Gottesman Library, founded in 1955, is the primary bibliographic resource facility serving the information needs of the AECOM and the Ferkauf Graduate School of Psychology of Yeshiva University. Used by an estimated 10,000 persons each year, the Library's collections consist of 74,890 monographic volumes and 2,736 current serial titles as well as special collections: history of medicine, archives, reference, and audiovisuals. In addition to serving this primary clientele, the Library supports the clinical and educational affiliations which the AECOM maintains with a number of hospital medical centers including the MMC.

Library Collaboration Agreement

In 1987 the MMC and AECOM, acting on recommendations outlined in a site visit report commissioned by the MMC, began the necessary legal and administrative negotiations required for collaboration and sharing of the library facilities of the two institutions. The report succinctly summarized the purpose of the consultation: "to identify the major planning issues and likely resources needed to achieve a state-of-the art medical literature and information delivery system."[1] Consequently, the medical library, renamed the Tishman Learning Center (TLC)[2] and opened in 1988, was designed with specifications to accommodate the installation and implementation of new information technologies. As envisioned by the MMC administration and the learning center designers, application of modern technologies included establishing a telecommunications link between the libraries of the MMC and the AECOM to facilitate the sharing of resources. This vision included the development of a microcomputer laboratory providing individual workstations equipped with a variety of popular software including word processing, database management, and spreadsheet programs. In addition, it was assumed that online clinical computer applications could be made available at these workstations as these programs were implemented. "This view incorporated the belief that libraries should no longer be viewed as physical places (rooms or buildings filled with books, journals, and other learning or study facilities), but serve as distributed sources of information and knowledge."[3] The consultants emphasized that newer technologies permit an escape from the confines of limiting physical structures. MMC was fortunate to purchase the expert, professional advice of outside consultants who "customed-tailored" their report to the MMC scene. However, much of this technical advice is also available in a general way in the literature. For example, what the librarian needs to know about building and constructing a computer room; linking separate physical locations by telecommunications, local area networks (LANs), and networks; installing and cabling terminals and the seemingly endless demands for electrical power sources have been summarized by Epstein.[4]

MMC Management Information System Specifications

The MMC Management Information System (MIS) group planned, prepared, and executed the technical specifications which included a broadband telecommunications system electronically linking the MMC and AECOM facilities. The MIS department oversaw the specifications and installation of all other computer peripherals in the TLC such as cabling units, telephone lines, communication jacks for personal computers, workstations, printers, and modems. Figure 1 shows the connectivity for the TLC as established on the MMC LAN utilizing the CATV cable system and broadband radio frequency modulation (FM from Hughes LAN System, formerly Sytek). The Center has its own subLAN employing a unique bandwidth over the FM spectrum. The communications software is NetWare/6000, an adaptation of Novell's Advanced NetWare Network Operating System (ANWNOS), with multitasking functionality, sharing of resources, and full support of NETBIOS standard. Security is provided down to the level of physical record locking. Additional features of this LAN connectivity are described below.

PC Server

The PC server function is provided with a Sytek PC, an Intel 80386 processor, with 32-bit transfer and a 180MB unformatted hard disk. Any PC connected to the TLC can share the hard disk and any future peripherals on the server. The recommended standard for attached devices is any IBM or IBM compatible PCs (286 processor or higher).

InterNetwork Bridge

This bridge, with its stand-alone hardware and software SyTerm, allows microcomputers in the TLC to connect to any host or terminal attached to the primary LAN. File transfer and terminal emulation of a wide range of standard ASCII terminal types are supported. The current specification of the hardware permits sixteen simultaneous sessions. Each additional connected PC will require a Network Adapter Card.

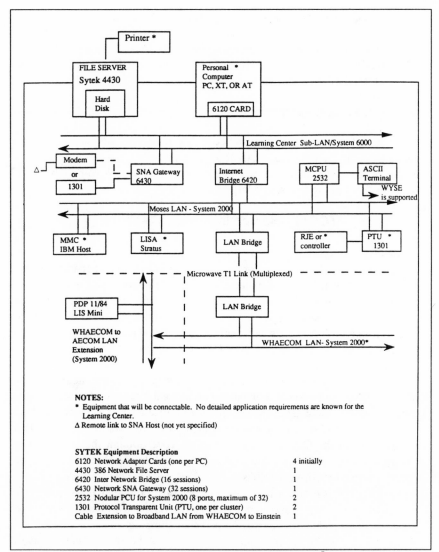

Figure 1. Topology of the connectivities in the Learning Center[5]

SNA Gateway

The gateway includes hardware and software for PCs in the TLC to link to any SNA network as an SNA type 1 or 2 logical unit. The current specifications support a maximum of thirty-two concurrent sessions with a single "hot" button to switch between an SNA application and DOS with full file transfer capability. Maximum communications speed is up to 19.2bps.

Direct Hookup with the Primary LAN

One Modular Packet Communication Unit (PCU) provides attachment of eight ASCII terminals to access any host connected to the primary LAN. The VT-100 standard is supported.

Future Enhancements

Additional PCUs can be installed with a modem so that remote users can connect to the System 6000 LAN through switch facilities. Additional hardware can be added to bridge the System 6000 into other Novell's ANWNOS systems functioning as a single large system.

AECOM Research Information Technology

Computing facilities for faculty research and student use at the AECOM are provided by the Research Information Technology (RIT) department. The RIT's activities involve computers and related electronic technologies. The RIT operates three VAX/Unix systems that provide twenty-four-hour time-sharing service. There are numerous dial-in terminal ports and three public-access rooms with terminals, personal computers, and related equipment on the AECOM campus. To date, no AECOM RIT equipment or service has ever been placed at the MMC.

Some of the main uses of time-shared computing at the medical school include DNA and protein sequencing, statistical analysis of research data, maintenance of databases, for example for clinical trials, electronic mail and news access, and word processing. Batch jobs are submitted to the IBM mainframes at the City University of New York through the Unix system. There is heavy reliance on software packages. All time-sharing services are provided on a fee-for-service basis.

The RIT operates a public-access personal computer room jointly for AECOM Gottesman Library and Yeshiva University MIS department which offers short introductory courses on personal computer topics such as Word-Perfect, Lotus, DOS, for example. Personal computers are also available in the Library's public terminal rooms where they are set up to communicate with the Unix systems including the library databases.

Unlike some other leading medical schools, AECOM and MMC are not affiliated with a major research university which can serve as a source for computer facilities and technical support or that can provide an organizational model for information technology services.

Shared Integration MMC-AECOM Library Resources

Negotiations are underway to install a full-fledged network between MMC and AECOM. However, the concept of shared integration of library resources began when the AECOM Gottesman Library and the MMC TLC agreed to establish mutually, shared responsibilities through contractual arrangements for an integrated library system. With this agreement in place, the MMC and AECOM selected the Georgetown University™ Library Information System (LIS), developed by the Dahlgren Memorial Library, as the automated library system of choice. LIS is nationally recognized as the leading health sciences library system. It is a comprehensive, integrated library system with networking features and applications that effectively include all library operations.[6]

Design of LIS

The LIS is briefly and best described in the following paragraphs taken from the LIS manual:

> As an integrated system, the LIS is composed of modules that share master files. The master bibliographic (MARC) file, the most important of the shared files, includes a single record for each book and journal title held by the library, as well as for those on-order and in-processing. This record is referenced by the online catalog for searching, by the circulation system for inventory control, and by the serials control system. Records for titles of new acquisitions are added to the master bibliographic file when items are ordered. The patron and item files function similarly, providing systematic control of all library functions.
>
> The LIS uses the standard MARC record format as the basis for its master bibliographic file. The system follows NLM [National Library of Medicine] or LC classification systems and can interface with NLM Medical Subject Headings (MeSH), ensuring standardization of subject terms in the Online Catalog and the miniMEDLINE SYSTEM™.
>
> The system can be adapted to meet the needs of most medical and other special libraries since its design allows for profiling such variables as circulation policies, MARC cataloging profiles, online cataloging help screens, circulation notices, and acquisitions policies without modifying the software.[7]

LIS is designed to function on minicomputer and microcomputer workstations. LIS can be adapted to a multiple library environment with dial-up access through a LAN. At MMC-AECOM, LIS operates on a DEC PDP 11/84 running the InterSystems MII+ MUMPS operating system.

Implementation of LIS

In 1987, the three major participants—MMC, AECOM, and Georgetown—signed a contract to begin the implementation of LIS at the MMC-AECOM sites. A project director was appointed to prepare the specifications, purchase the equipment and software, follow up on the renovation of the computer room and requisite air conditioning, and to begin training on the technical requirements of installing the system under the supervision of the Georgetown University Dahlgren Library LIS staff. The first LIS implementation and overview meeting held at AECOM in September 1987 was attended by nearly fifteen representatives from AECOM, MMC, and Georgetown.

During 1987–88, the LIS system was fully implemented at the host library (i.e., the Gottesman Library). When that was accomplished, the same procedures were implemented at the satellite MMC (TLC) Library. The libraries were set up to share a single master bibliographic file, while maintaining their own patron and item files. Users can search the catalogs of each library separately or as a combined union catalog. By 1991, the Georgetown LIS programming staff added a Document Delivery System (DDS) which permits patrons to request items online. Patrons can pick up items or have them sent by a fax machine or mailed. Requested items not found in the library's holdings may be requested by interlibrary loan. The DDS interacts with miniMEDLINE™ and the online catalog.

It had already been established that the miniMEDLINE module would be the first LIS function to be implemented so that both sites could use, share, and benefit from the bibliographic system. After the preparation of the computer room, installation of the PDP minicomputer with its attendant cabling and terminal setups, loading of the MII+ operating system, and loading of the appropriate LIS software, reading of the NLM MEDLINE tapes could begin. In this process citations from preselected MEDLINE titles are read and indexed in the computer's memory. With the miniMEDLINE database in place, patron access to this subset of NLM's MEDLINE database was made available to the MMC-AECOM communities on the May 15, 1988. The miniMEDLINE contains citations from 345 journals selected jointly by the libraries and is updated monthly.

To conduct a bibliographic search, users build sets of references by accessing author, title, journal, or subject files. The miniMEDLINE has Boolean AND/OR searching capabilities. Lists of references and abstracts can be stored in the patron's miniMEDLINE online file or printed online in alphabetical order by journal title.

While the preparations for the miniMEDLINE functionality were underway, related patron files were being created directly into the LIS. The system is also equipped to accept tape readable patron files when these tapes are available.

The creation of the LIS MARC catalog database was undertaken simultaneously through a contract with the PALINET OCLC network. The two libraries' online cataloging records were merged into a single database. These merged tapes were then encoded with MUMPS by the Georgetown LIS staff and the tape made ready for local tape loading.

After the loading of the processed cataloging database, barcode linking of catalog and serial records to individual LIS MARC items was begun. This process was the single most time-consuming project as the library holdings, monographic and serial, were brought one by one into the LIS system in anticipation of online circulation procedures. The LIS circulation module features: check-out, check-in, renew, hold, and recall functions. It also alerts users to inappropriate transactions, fines and overdues, and generates patron overdue notices.

The LIS designates the host site (AECOM) as the cataloging site. The cataloging workflow including authority file maintenance between the two libraries has been determined by administrative agreement which includes routines to be followed, plus the personnel and budgetary arrangements. The LIS cataloging utilities function allows the professional staff to create, edit, and store bibliographic records in full MARC format. It interfaces with NLM MeSH, unlike many other automated library systems,[8] and allows downloading from the OCLC database to the LIS database.

The LIS online catalog allows users to search all the library's holdings using the standard access points: author, title, keyword, and subject. Users may view and print a catalog display that replicates a standard catalog card, determine the item's status (available, on loan, etc.), and see where it is located in the library.

The MMC-AECOM libraries learned that modernized services place added strains on all library staff. This is especially true during the difficult crossover period when old, manual routines are still in place, but one is trying to implement the new, computerized routines which staff are trying to learn. We found that taking the leap to the new system as quickly as possible worked best for us.

The LIS has a variety of management reports available in each of its modules which allow continuous, updated management records of the library to be generated. Patron usage of the miniMEDLINE SYSTEM is carefully monitored using the report mechanisms. Similarly, LIS reports in each of the other LIS modules provide up-to-date financial accounting from acquisitions, and item location status reports from the acquisitions, serials, and cataloging modules. Circulation reports include monitoring of hourly patron usage of this function which helps in scheduling staff at the circulation desk.

Conclusion and Future Plans

By implementing LIS using a partnering approach the two libraries have benefited and more than complied with the recommendations of the MMC consultant team. The consultants wrote of their belief that the information requirements for modern medical care delivery organizations rest on three simple principles:[9]

1. Health professionals, during the course of their work, must have easy access to multiple sources of high-quality information pertinent to their work.
2. Easy access to multiple sources of information requires electronic networks that permit access from any worksite to different types of files and databases located both on and off the premises.
3. The information environment of a medical center must be carefully designed with the two foregoing principles in mind and managed by the senior administrator who can assign the appropriate priority for attention and resources.

The shared MMC-AECOM library system project called for a high level of cooperation between the two libraries and their staffs. In addition, the Georgetown LIS staff provided generous and unlimited encouragement, advice, and assistance in implementing the LIS system. As we learn to share the unity of our two libraries on an ongoing basis, the LIS has remained the common functionality which builds a highly useful bridge.

With this shared bibliographic foundation in place, it is hoped future commitments to medical informatics of the kind described by Broering[10] can be brought to actuality for researchers and clinicians at the TLC. These include online access to patient records, verification of diagnostic findings, drug protocols, medical models and simulations, as well as access to and exchange of traditional and non-traditional bibliographic data in an electronic environment. The MMC is beginning to plan an extension of the Library's information technology activities into these areas.

References

1. Nina Matheson, Edward H. Shortliffe, and Marjorie P. Wilson, "The Robert and Phyllis Tishman Learning Center: site visit report," (January 1987). Unpublished, p. 3.

2. Debra C. Rand, MMC librarian from 1982 to 1987 was largely responsible for the design of the Tishman Learning Center.
3. Matheson, Shortliffe, and Wilson, p. 5.
4. Susan Baerg Epstein, "Automation dreams versus reality," *Library Journal* (September 15, 1986): 48–49; and Susan Baerg Epstein, "Automation takes longer than you planned," *Library Journal* (May 15, 1986): 48–49.
5. Ron Lei, "LAN connectivity specifications at the Robert and Phyllis Tishman Learning Center, MMC" (1987). Unpublished.
6. Naomi C. Broering, "The Georgetown University Library Information System (LIS): a minicomputer-based integrated library system," *Bulletin of the Medical Library Association* 71 (July 1983): 317–23; and Naomi C. Broering, "An affordable microcomputer library information system developed by Georgetown University," *Microcomputers for Information Management* 1 (December 1984): 269–83; and Naomi C. Broering and Cannard Bonnie, "Building bridges: LIS-IAIMS BioSYNTHESIS," *Special Libraries* 79 (Fall 1988): 302–13.
7. *The Library Information System, Version 4.3 User Guide*, Vol. 1 (Library Computer Services: Dahlgren Memorial Library, Georgetown University Medical Center, August 15, 1990), A–4.
8. Sarah Hager Johnston, "Desperately seeking authority control: automated systems are not providing it," *Library Journal* (October 1, 1990): 43–46.
9. Matheson, Shortliffe, and Wilson, p. 5.
10. Naomi C. Broering, "MAClinical workstation project at Georgetown University," *Bulletin of the Medical Library Association* 79 (July 1991): 276–81.

CHAPTER 13.
INTEGRATION AND BEYOND AT THE UPJOHN PHARMACEUTICAL LIBRARY

June E. Hauck
Information Scientist
Corporate Technical Library
The Upjohn Company

Abstract

The Upjohn Company Corporate Technical Library is a research-based technical library with a mission of supporting Upjohn's worldwide pharmaceutical businesses with access to technical information, management of internal information, and technical information products and services. In 1991, the Library was organized into market-based product support teams in order to meet its goals of simplifying information access; compressing time lines for processes, products, and services; and improving its performance. This case study provides a snapshot of a technology-based, customer-driven corporate library as it moves towards its vision of becoming an online library providing desktop access to value-added information for informed decisions.

Introduction

The Upjohn Company is a worldwide, research-based producer and marketer of pharmaceuticals, fine chemicals, and seed and agricultural specialties. Kalamazoo, Michigan, serves as the corporate, research, and medical headquarters, and the home of its domestic pharmaceutical manufacturing organization. There are 20,000 Upjohn employees worldwide, approximately 8,000 in the Kalamazoo area, including 1,200 research division (Upjohn Laboratories) personnel. Library information services are provided by the Corporate Technical Library (CTL), the Business Library, and Medical Library Services, which serves the clinical development and medical affairs areas. A number of unit (departmental) collections in Kalamazoo, plus overseas collections and information services, form an Upjohn Library network. The CTL has a regular full-time staff of thirty (sixteen library information professionals and fourteen office support staff) plus a number of part-time and temporary staff. The mission of the Library is to support the goals and strategies of Upjohn's worldwide pharmaceutical and related businesses by providing timely access to technical information, cost-effective management of internal information, and value-added technical information products and services.

Library Services

In addition to technical and information services common to most libraries, the CTL has responsibility for several corporate information systems. Library staff create and maintain the corporate Product Information Retrieval System/ Upjohn (PIRSU) database and a published product literature archive. PIRSU is searchable online from any Upjohn location worldwide. A parallel online information system for internal proprietary literature (TREK: Technical Reports Electronic Knowledgebase) is also created and maintained by library staff.

The Library is open twenty-four hours for company walk-in customers, but is staffed only for the normal eight-hour workday. A large portion of the customer population, especially those offsite and overseas, access library services through telephone, fax, mail, and electronic means. Library information specialists and information scientists with degrees in both the chemical or biological sciences and library/information science, provide reference services, literature search services, and current literature alerting. Customer education programs include library seminars, tours and orientations for individuals or groups, instruction for specific subject area resources, and end-user online search training.

All technical services operations—acquisitions, serials control, bindery, cataloging—are supported by the LIS (Library Information System), an integrated library automation system. The CTL is the central cataloging unit for all Upjohn libraries and unit collections. A corporate online catalog is supported by LIS, as is automated circulation of library materials. Document delivery services are also provided.

Library Collection

The size of the collection, especially the retention of bound periodicals (82,000 volumes), is a reflection of the geographic location of the library and the need to provide rapid turnaround on document requests. There are no nearby major medical, scientific, or technical library resources for local document delivery backup. Although a library devoted primarily to current research, the CTL has nevertheless kept a rather large number of older periodicals. This is changing as new technologies for electronic transmission and production of full text make keeping large collections less and less cost effective. A document delivery volume of 40,000 copies per year including 15,000 requests from outside sources and an annual circulation of 10,000 reflect these changes.

Special attention to collection control, not just development, is still critical in this environment. The collection is reviewed annually for retention and discard decisions. Product literature, technical reports, patents, and some periodical indexes are kept either on 16mm microfilm cartridges or on optical disk. A weekly library publication (available both online and in paper form) announces additions to the CTL, including videotapes of in-house lectures and presentations from invited speakers, plus additions to the decentralized unit collections.

The Library Vision: Towards the "Virtual Library"

As we entered the 1990s, it became increasingly obvious that corporate libraries needed a new approach to help their parent companies stay competitive in an age of global expansion coupled with downsizing. Instead of simply using technology as a productivity tool to automate routine manual tasks, we needed to look at ways that technology could expand the physical limits of both the library and the staff. Expanding the services of the library beyond the physical boundaries has been described as the "virtual library."[1] It is central to CTL's vision to provide interactive, desktop access to value-added information products and services. This means providing electronic access to customers located on the next floor or on the next continent. It also means providing access to information resources within the library, within the corporation and within the world, as if these resources were all located in the same room.

To be considered a valuable company asset, the corporate library must be perceived as progressive, proactive, responsive, flexible, and able to respond rapidly to changing priorities. Library services and library staff must be visibly supporting priority corporate programs. To achieve this vision, in 1991 the CTL was reorganized from the traditional "information services" and "technical services" departmental structure to a new structure consisting of teams designated to support CTL products and services. All CTL staff involved in the development, maintenance, production, or provision of a library product or service were named as participants in the team for that product. Each team has responsibility for planning, developing, maintaining, improving, promoting, supporting, or eliminating a product. Using the CTL mission and goals as a framework, the teams develop product marketing strategies. These strategies help determine how the team will move on a particular product, and they rely on an ongoing market research effort involving continuous customer contact and feedback. From the product strategy, the teams develop objectives and goals, and these are then translated into individual action plans and incorporated into performance goals for each team member.

Library management provided team operating guidelines, lists of team members, and named the initial team leaders and facilitators. Several days of training launched the teams and periodic training or development assistance is provided to teams and/or individuals. Training covers topics such as how to work together as a team, team operations, solving interpersonal conflicts, communications, and problem solving. A staff development team monitors the progress of the teams and checks for further training needs. Library staff and management feel that the market-oriented approach to library services will make the CTL products and services more sensitive to customer and business needs. Also, the team approach will do a great deal to enhance staff development, empower individuals, and free them to contribute even greater creativity and commitment to the success of the Library and of The Upjohn Company.

Collection Resources Team and the Cataloging Team

The collection resources team and the cataloging team are designed to organize and provide bibliographic access to materials held in The Upjohn Company libraries and selected collections, and to provide consultation services for organization and access to other company materials.

Since 1984, the CTL has used Georgetown University's™ LIS to automate the familiar library functions of circulation, acquisitions, cataloging, serials control, and bindery, and to provide a corporatewide Upjohn Libraries Online Catalog. The system runs on a DEC VAX 6210 attached to the company's local area network (LAN). Any library customer worldwide whose workstation is connected to the LAN network can search the corporate catalog. In addition, software resident on the Upjohn Laboratories IBM 3090 mainframe allows the 1,500 worldwide users of that computer to "pass through" to the VAX 6210 in order to search the catalog. This electronic access to the contents of all Upjohn libraries constitutes a virtual library for Upjohn employees around the world. Customers may easily search the holdings of all Upjohn libraries and unit collections from their workstations or from secure dial-up access to the company network.

Part of the vision of the CTL is to expand the library integrated system beyond the basic collection control functions to serve as a library resource management tool. We anticipate increases in electronic connections to library vendors: bibliographic utilities, serial subscription agencies, and publishers. The goal will be to promote as much as possible the interchange of information in electronic form between the corporate library and its vendors. This could include use of information already provided by publishers, such as barcodes on periodical issues. The online catalog, too, can be expanded in many ways beyond its traditional boundaries. Not only will we consider the inclusion of more types of materials in the catalog, but also an expansion of the catalog record itself to contain more detailed content information (tables of contents, chapter headings, etc.). Another expansion would result in a catalog that would be interactive with customers, allowing them to dynamically make requests, holds, purchase suggestions, and other comments. Items requested electronically can be pulled by library staff and mailed to the requester's location, resulting in a productive use of time for all concerned.

Circulation/Document Delivery Team

The CTL's document delivery area handles a volume of approximately 40,000 photocopy and ILL requests per year. Customers may submit requests on standard multipart request forms by fax, electronic forms, e-mail messages, or by submitting copies of literature searches or published bibliographies with the desired citation highlighted or circled. Copies that can be provided from the CTL's collection are furnished free, while copies that must be acquired outside, and "rush" copies are charged back to the requester's unit. The Library strives to achieve twenty-four-hour turnaround on requests for items held locally. Requests received on electronic forms (about one-third of the total) are stored online so that they may be analyzed by many data points. Non-electronic requests have only the requester's name and unit number keyed into the system, so that we may generate rudimentary statistics. Many copies are purchased from document vendors, reflecting the frequent need for rapid delivery of information over the lower cost of interlibrary loans.

The use of document vendors and interlibrary loans presents to the customer another view of the virtual library: that through one source they can get a copy of nearly any published material needed for their work. Document delivery staff are able to virtually "pull from the shelves" items from the world's knowledge base. But much of the daily work in this area is paper-based. To achieve our vision of the next-generation document delivery system, we need to target improvements. For example, our present electronic document request form is simply an online version of the paper request form, and the customer just keys in the citation instead of writing it. We plan links so that a customer searching a literature database available on the Upjohn network (e.g., Current Contents on Diskette®) will simply flag the citations of interest and they will be automatically forwarded to the library along with the customer's name, address and phone number (captured electronically). We will be able to pre-flag citations in the database to indicate those sources held by the local library. This will assist customers who wish to make their own copies from the library's collection.

Another enhancement involves providing customers with literature search results from outside databases in electronic form. The electronic bibliography will be processed before being sent to the customer, to flag the items held locally. The customer will then receive and view the search results using specially developed software so that they may selectively send items from the list back to the library for copy acquisition. The citation will be captured in its entirety and will not need to be rekeyed and hence mistyped. Document delivery software at the library's end will manage the electronic requests, allowing them to be easily sorted, printed, queried, and summarized. Requests which must be purchased from outside may be electronically forwarded to our document vendor, while being automatically logged and tracked in our own database. Data will be readily available for copyright and collection development needs. And, cost reports can be generated for unit management if request costs need to be charged back.

Literature Research Team and the Reference Services Team

The literature research team and the reference services team provide literature and information to support Upjohn research and development. They assist library users in the identification and location of needed information through the direct provision of user assistance and the development and maintenance of related library collections.

A staff of library information specialists and information scientists provides literature research and reference service for customers. An average of 2,500 literature search requests are handled each year, and some 1,000 current alerting profiles are maintained for 700 subscribers. Customers request literature searches in person, through a paper form, an online electronic form, and over the telephone. Searches are conducted using Crosstalk telecommunications software and modems that are part of the Upjohn telephone system. The Library also leases a direct high-speed line to BRS Information Technologies, and any BRS databases may be searched over this line from the Upjohn Laboratories IBM mainframe without incurring telecommunications charges. Search results are either printed directly or downloaded into WordPerfect 5.1 where they may be edited and augmented with the addition of highlighting, headers, footers, and cover sheets. Records of each literature search request are maintained in an online log which allows us to track how quickly the search is moving through the cycle and how often we meet or exceed the requester's due date.

Most current alerting profiles are stored with the vendor and run monthly. Resulting printouts are mailed to the Library where they are distributed by CTL staff to the various subscribers. Some current alerting is also run in-house with locally developed software and purchased tapes of bibliographic citations. These alerts are printed in-house on laser printers and distributed using interoffice mail. The Library also conducts several classes per year on searching Chemical Abstracts, MEDLINE, and the company's internal databases PIRSU and TREK. We train between 200 and 300 end-users each year.

As part of our vision for literature research services, we will be providing more information in electronic form. Literature search results will be more often sent electronically over the network or the mainframe so that the customer may review the output online and easily request copies or further information. Current alerts will also be provided electronically instead of in printed form, and will be distributed as electronic mail to subscribers. By participating directly in drug development teams, library staff will be expanding on the CTL's proactive approach to information services by developing an understanding of what is important to the customer, gaining new knowledge of how information is used in scientific research, and creating customized products and services to suit the preferences of targeted customers. Our goal is to be a valuable part of the research team working to develop drugs.

TREK Team

The TREK (Technical Reports Electronic Knowledgebase) team is designed to provide access to proprietary technical information.

TREK is a database containing proprietary technical information that is maintained by CTL staff. The TREK team manages the database and the associated document archive. The database at present contains 30,000 citations to internal technical documents including abstracts and indexer-assigned keywords chosen from an online technical thesaurus also maintained by the team. The online record points to the complete text of the document. Before 1991, documents were stored on microfilm cartridges. More recent documents are available on an optical disk system. The staff members of the TREK team have responsibility for receiving technical documents from various divisions of the company, scanning them onto optical disk, and indexing them. The Library also receives an electronic copy of the title page, which is used as the basis for the citation that appears in the database. The indexer keywords and other information are added later. The database is available on the Upjohn Laboratories IBM 3090 mainframe under the STAIRS text storage and retrieval software and may be searched by Upjohn employees around the world. A security scheme ensures that only authorized employees are allowed access to TREK.

Concerning TREK, the Library envisions many changes in the early 1990s. One change is emerging from the desire to reduce human intellectual resources dedicated to indexing technical documents. New software is being proposed by the Library which will enable us to create a database containing the full text of the documents searchable by each word. In addition, the technical thesaurus presently maintained by the TREK team will be incorporated into a rich vocabulary permitting retrieval by concepts. Customers will be able to enter their information requirements in English sentences and the software will parse the request into its component concepts and retrieve the most relevant documents matching the query. This type of "concept-based" software will take us beyond the traditional inverted index full-text database and allow easy, accurate retrieval of complex queries as well as more rudimentary author, date, and compound queries.

Another aspect of the vision is the ability to send electronic text and images to requesters through the company network. Customers will be able to retrieve the full text of a document from the database and receive a WordPerfect 5.1 file containing the text. Further down the road, we anticipate network links to the optical disk system so that customers may retrieve a document ID from the database and request an electronic image from optical disk which would contain the graphical information unable to appear in the database. Besides giving customers access to the virtual library of Upjohn technical documents, the new generation TREK will also reduce the time needed to make information available.

PIRSU Team

The PIRSU team provides published product literature information to meet the research, regulatory, and medical monitoring requirements of the worldwide pharmaceutical and agricultural businesses.

PIRSU (Product Information Retrieval System/Upjohn) is the company's database containing published literature about Upjohn products and product candidates. The PIRSU team is responsible for maintaining the database and its associated literature archive. The team maintains search profiles with several database vendors, which result in regular electronic shipments of new literature citations discussing Upjohn products. Photocopies are acquired for each article and they are sent in batches to outside indexing agencies where they are evaluated for relevancy. The articles designated as "in scope" are indexed according to a library-provided thesaurus. The electronic citations with indexing terms are returned along with the hard copies. The citations are added to the PIRSU database, a private file on the BRS system. The photocopies are scanned into the optical disk system from which high-quality copies may be obtained rapidly. Articles before 1991 are available on microfilm cartridges. There is an active program to train interested Upjohn employees to search PIRSU, and over 300 employees have BRS ID codes for this purpose.

The CTL vision for product literature management will also depend on new text management software. The task of tracking product literature citations from their receipt through copy ordering, copy receipt, transmittal to indexing agencies, return from the indexers, editing, scanning onto optical disk, and finally, addition to the database, is intricate and requires flexible text database management software with good report-generating capabilities. In addition, the accompanying thesaurus needs to be available in a database so that terms and "see references" may be easily added and used to validate the indexing terms assigned to new citations entering the database.

The "concept-based" text retrieval software proposed for the TREK database is also a potential solution for product literature retrieval. At present the

PIRSU thesaurus is a paper tool which searchers consult to select the most appropriate terms for their query. There is no capability for the thesaurus to be an online tool unless we move the database to an in-house computer running comprehensive text management software. This possibility will be carefully analyzed by the team to determine the cost-effectiveness of such a move and to ensure that worldwide access by Upjohn subsidiaries would be maintained at the same level. Our vision for text software will include electronic current alerts to subscribers who maintain their subject interest profiles with the Library. Eventually, customers searching the PIRSU database will be able to send requests for particular articles across the network to the optical disk system and receive the image back at their workstations.

Access to Published Literature Databases

To provide better service to customers and to fulfill customer needs for fast access to published literature and information, the Library vision includes the creation of more in-house databases of published literature. Our first venture into this area was loading the Current Contents on Diskette (CCoD) software on the network and making it available to all employees with access to the network. The Library maintains the database by loading new issues of CCoD as they arrive and deleting old issues. Customers are able to easily search for information themselves or to store profiles of their subject interests to run against new issues as they arrive. Citations of interest may be saved to an electronic file and forwarded to the Library's document delivery area. The networked CCoD service has been requested strongly by customers and can result in a significant savings by the cancellation of subscriptions to the paper product.

With new text storage, retrieval and management software available, the Library will look carefully at providing in-house access to other literature databases for both end-user searching and current alerting. Locally developed software that provides paper current alerts from purchased tapes of literature citations would be a good candidate for replacement by new software. Increased flexibility, easy end-user menu-based searching, electronic alerting, and electronic forwarding of document requests are all features that we envision and that will make the proposed systems more productive for the customer. Library customers are increasingly interested in searching the literature themselves, and providing them an easy and cost-effective way to do this is a vital part of the Library's mission.

Library Systems Team

The library systems team provides operations support, data processing, systems analysis, training, and troubleshooting for CTL staff and other library automation users within Upjohn data security guidelines and practices, and provides consulting and support services for information storage and retrieval projects to all Upjohn personnel as requested.

The library systems team has responsibility for maintaining all library computer systems and equipment and so acts as a service unit to the staff of the library. Systems support is provided during all aspects of a particular project, from systems analysis and definition of project requirements, to software recommendation and selection, customized programming or support for "off-the-shelf" products, system development and testing, ongoing maintenance, and troubleshooting and problem resolution. In addition, the team has responsibility for administering the library's capital budget, recommending and ordering equipment, overseeing installation and testing, and ongoing support. Telecommunications support also comes under the area of the systems team, and the team acts as a liaison to outside vendors and to other computer and telecommunications areas of the Company.

Because the systems team is charged with supporting all library computer projects, it has knowledge and expertise in every area of the library. Some of the projects that the team has developed offer an opportunity to "tie together" the various library products and services and provide a centralized source of information for customers. The most visible project, the Library Gateway System, is available to the 1,500 users of the Upjohn Laboratories IBM 3090 mainframe and serves as a central access point for most library services. A menu-based, function key-driven program guides the user to the service options. The user's name, company address, and phone number are automatically captured and forwarded to the library along with any requests made. All activity on the gateway is logged so that transactions may be analyzed to determine which services might be added or deleted from the menus. A central menu guides the user to a choice of either searching one of the library's databases, sending a request to the library, or viewing information provided by the library.

When the user selects the option to search a library database, he/she is presented with a secondary menu that lists the databases available. If the user selects to search the company's online library catalog, he/she is passed to the LIS online catalog on the CTL's VAX 6210. When the search is completed, a function key returns the user to the gateway menu. If the user selects to search the PIRSU database, he/she must have a BRS ID code and have some knowledge of log-on and searching techniques. Those with BRS ID codes are passed to the BRS computer via the library's dedicated high-speed connection. The user may send prints to a local mainframe printer or may capture screens of information to a file on their mainframe ID. Upon logging off, the user is returned to the same gateway menu. Other database choices on this menu send the user to the TREK database on STAIRS and to other, smaller STAIRS databases maintained by the library. When the new text software is installed, the gateway will allow users to search databases on that software using a menu and function key-based search screen.

Upon selecting the gateway option to send a request to the library, the user sees a secondary menu listing the various types of requests he/she can send. Each type of request pulls up a different online electronic form which is filled in by the user and then electronically forwarded to the library. Users may send photocopy or document delivery requests, requests for copies of PIRSU articles, technical document copy requests, reference questions or suggestions, and literature search requests. If the user elects to send an electronic literature search request, the user can further designate whether he/she wants to send it to a particular information specialist or scientist, or just to send it to any available searcher. This gateway menu also allows the user to add or delete his/her name from the library's mailing list, and to send an electronic form listing news about upcoming seminars or lectures. The latter events are included in an online and print publication produced by the library entitled *Events of Research Interest*.

A third option on the gateway main menu lets the user view the latest information from the library. A secondary menu displays several types of information available for viewing. Users can see a list of the most recent technical reports received by the library for processing into the TREK database. A brief citation to the technical report is displayed on the screen, and the user may strike function keys to print it or to order a copy of the full report. Another file available for viewing is a list of the most recent additions to the library collection (a "new book" list). These items are grouped by broad subject categories (biology, chemistry, pharmacology, etc.) and each book on the list is assigned a function key. Striking the function key next to a book title results in a request for that book being sent to the library. The library staff either pulls the book and mails it to the requester, or puts the requester's name on a hold list for that book. Users can also view a list of journal issues checked in over the past ten days. Many library customers like to scan new issues of their favorite journals when they arrive, and this list is an easy way to tell when the next issue has been received. The list is generated from the LIS system. Finally, users may view a list of upcoming events of research interest, including seminars and lectures by outside speakers.

All requests generated by the gateway system are sent to a central library ID on the IBM mainframe computer. Several times a day, a staff member logs on to the central ID and retrieves all the accumulated requests. A program sorts the requests by type, and either prints them or forwards them to the appropriate staff member to handle. Detailed transaction logs are kept so that requests can be analyzed by type, by customer, by the requester's unit, and by broad divisions of the company.

The gateway service is one of the newest offered by the library. But it is far from complete. We have a vision of a far more comprehensive system acting as the entry for all customers of electronic information products and services. As new databases are added to the library's text management software, they will be incorporated onto the gateway menus to achieve the broadest possible usage. We envision the customer being able to set up a current alerting profile through the gateway, and to receive their regular alerts individually directed to them. We want to add more "bulletin board" type information so that announcements of upcoming library classes or new services can be widely advertised. We envision replacing our present printed newsletter with an online version viewable through the gateway. We plan to add other Upjohn libraries to the system so that requests would be sent to the library nearest the customer, based on their address. And finally, we want to be compatible with future computing directions by moving the system from the IBM mainframe to the company network where it would have a wider client base. Library databases and applications being mounted on the network could then be easily included in the gateway menus. This would go far towards presenting the library customer with their own virtual library of services from one central menu.

Conclusion

The Corporate Technical Library has made great strides towards its vision of becoming an online library providing desktop access to value-added information for informed decisions. To make further progress towards the goal, the staff must be able to manage library resources in an effective manner that focuses on company and divisional priorities, while simplifying information access for the customer and compressing the time lines for library processes, products, and services. The image projected by the Library and its staff must be that of a progressive, proactive, responsive, and flexible team player, perceived by upper management and by customers as a valuable company asset, and perceived by our colleagues as a leader in information vision and planning. Fostering a team environment that promotes personal growth will allow our staff to focus on achieving new heights in customer service. Providing the virtual library for our customers will help us achieve our goals and continuously improve our products, services, and image. To succeed in the next decade will require nothing less.

Reference

1. M. Mitchell and L. M. Saunders, "The virtual library: an agenda for the 1990s," *Computers in Libraries* 11 (April 1991): 8, 10–11.

CHAPTER 14.
INFORMATION TECHNOLOGY AT
THE ROYAL COLLEGE OF PHYSICIANS
OF EDINBURGH LIBRARY

Iain A. Milne
Deputy Librarian
Royal College of Physicians of Edinburgh

Abstract

This chapter details library experiences with information technology in a small independently financed professional association—the Royal College of Physicians of Edinburgh. The College, its management structure, and computer history are discussed. Changes in the College library's market and the library staff's use of information technology to continue current information services in a difficult environment are described. Library involvement providing college-wide computer support is discussed. Plans to automate the catalogue are examined. The chapter concludes with some reflections on the College's information technology experience.

The Royal College of Physicians of Edinburgh

The Royal College of Physicians of Edinburgh (RCPE)* was granted a Royal Charter by King Charles II in 1681. The College is a United Kingdom professional association principally concerned with the maintenance of standards of postgraduate medical training and practice; the acquisition and dissemination of medical knowledge and the provision of medical advice to government, national bodies, and the public. The College is well known to many doctors who (at the end of their general professional training) sit through the Member of the Royal College of Physicians MRCP(UK), a searching theoretical and clinical examination which is jointly organised with the Royal Colleges in

---

* *The RCPE and College are used interchangeably throughout this paper for the Royal College of Physicians of Edinburgh.*

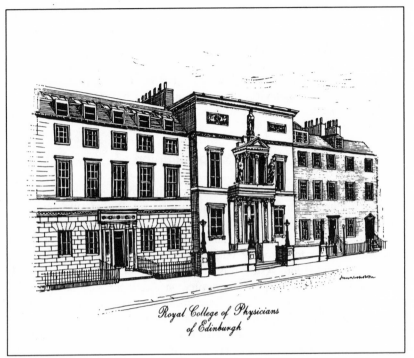

Figure 1. The Medical Library is located in the Royal College of Physicians.

Glasgow and London. Continuing medical education is another important college task, it holds lectures and symposia, publishes the journal *Proceedings of the Royal College of Physicians of Edinburgh,* and sponsors a research unit. The College has charitable status. It is not financed or controlled by government or other bodies.

The College (illustration shown in Figure 1) occupies four architecturally important buildings situated in central Edinburgh. No.8 Queen Street was built in 1770 as a domestic residence to the design of Robert Adam. No.9, first occupied in 1846, was built by Thomas Hamilton for the College. In 1876, David Bryce added the new library based on the layout of the Bodleian at Oxford. The College also owns No.11 Queen Street. Behind No.11 is a 300-seat conference centre. The College's premises provide a professional society with a prestigious home. They also provide reasonable storage for a large collection of books and journals. Unfortunately, the buildings were not designed for modern office work. Staff, who are distributed throughout the premises in inflexible rooms, feel that they are working in isolation. The organisation's splendid (if anachronistic) accommodation also makes siting and linking modern technology difficult and expensive.

The complex management structure of the RCPE can be compared to an elected government with a permanent civil service. The College's fellows elect a president and council who control the organisation through a network of committees. The average presidential term is three years. Although this system (which has been in existence for 300 years) has successfully preserved continuity, it restricts the scope of the organisation's full-time salaried executive. Checks and balances can cause problems when developing forward-looking plans or managing change.

RCPE's Computer History

The RCPE has a small staff. There are less than thirty salaried employees working in four departments. The workload is varied. During 1985 some employees (at various levels in the organisational hierarchy) felt it would be advantageous if certain manual procedures were automated. For instance, the library was anxious to introduce online searching, Administration wanted to automate the card record system used to record fellows' and members' details and the finance/appeals department desired an electronic accounting system. Advice was sought from a U.K. government body, the Common Services Agency. A consultant (with experience of the large database systems used by the Scottish Health Service) recommended a system and, after college council approval, two International Computers Limited (ICL) machines (based on the 8088 microprocessor) were purchased. Membership record work had been subcontracted to the Bank of Scotland. These records were retrieved and they formed the core of a RCPE records system based on the Dataflex multi-user database programme. This system grew "organically"; much of the work was done by an outside programmer. Although there was some ambivalence about the College's two ICL machines, they were successfully used for some word processing, accounts, automated direct debiting, mailing labels, and report generation.

In April 1987, a different management style was introduced following creation of the college manager, a new post established by the College Council. This was an attempt to end departmental isolation and provide a better link with the council. Shortly after this appointment, a new consultant (with a business background) was asked to investigate the organisation's use of computers. In Great Britain during this period there was spectacular growth in PC usage caused by the drop in hardware and software prices that followed the launch of the Amstrad 1,512 personal computer and other "clones" based on the IBM compatible Intel 8086 microprocessor. Many small organisations could now afford to use information technology. The RCPE took advantage of these developments; it bought a 20MB hard disk and twin floppy Amstrad 1640 PCs. Now more staff had access to PCs and they were able to use industry-standard spreadsheet, database, and word processor software to automate a wide variety of activities.

The Library and Its Market

The library, founded in 1682, was established by Sir Robert Sibbald, the principal founder of the College, and it has had a continuous existence as a working medical library since that date.[1] The library's many treasures include copies of the first editions of William Harvey's *De Motu Cordis* and Celsus' *De Medicina*. Three professional and two non-professional staff work in the library's three rooms in the main (nineteenth-century) part of the College's central Edinburgh buildings.

In the late 1980s, many professional associations (their finances threatened by a rising inflation rate and by the problems associated with the recruitment and retention of subscription-paying members) reexamined their operations. In this demanding environment hard-pressed finance committees questioned everything from accommodation to services. The RCPE did not escape examination. The library, an easily identified cost centre, was closely scrutinised and library staff had to develop new strategies to meet this challenge.

As college committees questioned the purpose of the library, marketing, with its customer/user orientation, became increasingly important to library staff. The marketing staff (influenced by works like Philip Kotler's frequently cited 1970's book extending the exchange concept to non-profit organisations) started to examine the library's market.[2] A grouping that includes the College's 3,000 fellows and 1,400 members, historians, and postgraduate students formed the primary market. The secondary market includes academics, the general public, genealogists, students, tourists, and other libraries. There is also an internal market—the library is regularly used by other college departments and provides information on a wide variety of topics; it is ultimately responsible for the Colleges' extensive administrative archives.

Investigations made it clear that the library was no longer a monopoly supplier of current medical information; it operated in a mature market to geographically widespread users. Although the subscription-paying membership of the College still made up the largest group of library users, many of the non-historical and archival services offered to them had been duplicated or superseded. Crucially, not all of the College's fellows and members made use of library' services. Some influential fellows had very little library contact. How could these opinion formers be persuaded that the library was contributing to the success of the College. It was clear that even the efficient provision of state-of-the-art library services would not alter some perceptions. The library's profile had to be raised with this important market grouping. The internal market offered one way to do this.

Library Information Technology Involvement

In 1992, Richard Smith wrote, "culturally librarians have stopped thinking of themselves as archivists and come to see themselves as information scientists."[3] The library staff in the RCPE certainly interpreted their role as information organisers and retrievers widely, and in 1988 college "computing" seemed a natural area for library input. Although anxious to become involved in the second wave of college-wide computerisation, they were initially unsure how they could best contribute. However, information technology had become integral to college operations and the library staff had quickly acquired the skills needed to use much of the IBM-compatible software on the new machines. As library expertise became known staff in other college departments started to ask them to solve their information technology (IT) problems. Although there were skilled members of staff in other departments, college computer users knew that the library enquiry desk was always staffed. They could get a quick response and often a quick solution to their enquiry or problem from there.

The system supported includes twenty PCs ranging from twin floppy Amstrad 8086 machines to IBM 386 PCs with large hard disks running under either MS DOS 3.2 or MS DOS 5. Microsoft Windows is available on two machines (see Figures 2 and 3). A wide variety of printers ranging from basic dot-matrix machines to Hewlett-Packard Laserjet IIIs are available. The College has also bought a variety of software packages. Many college information technology users just use the NewWord 2 word-processing package. New-

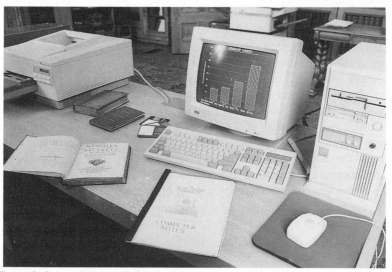

Figure 2. Computer workstations available for use in the library

Word is similar to WordStar and, during 1992, WordStar 7 was phased-in as a replacement. The SuperCalc 3 spreadsheet is used for budgets, reports and graphs. FormTool Gold is used to produce the college events sheet. The Ventura Desktop Publisher program is used for reports or documents which require special enhancement. For example, the college directory is produced by downloading dBase III records into Ventura. The finance department uses two modules of the Tetra 2000 accounting package—Nominal Ledger and Cash Book (which includes an automatic cheque writing facility). Pegasus Payroll is used to process all staff salaries. A recently introduced modem link to the Bank of Scotland HOBS system is used to carry out financial transactions. Dataflex has been replaced; fellows and members records are now organised on a dBase III program written for the College. This program runs on a Dell 286 in the finance department linked to an Amstrad in administration. Information is updated weekly and this allows reports to be produced in each department.

This link is unsatisfactory and the College is in the process of upgrading these machines and installing a small network to link them. Because of the importance of the membership and subscription data to most departments, installing a college network has often been given detailed consideration. However the integration of modern technology (especially long runs of computer cable) into eighteenth and nineteenth century buildings is difficult and expensive. Also, new departments are currently being created and this causes accommodation uncertainty. In the long term, networking seems inevitable and current library plans will make it more likely. The College is also considering the space-saving potential of scanners linked to optical storage devices.

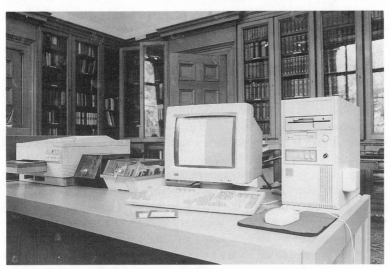

Figure 3. Computer workstations available for use in the library

As college in-house expertise increases and as the external environment continues to change, the library has tried to develop a coordinated IT plan. It has involved representatives from college departments in developing the following common aims:

1. Make less use of outside consultants.
2. Make more use of standard software.
3. Improve the presentation of college documents.
4. Upgrade to good quality, flexible, ergonomic equipment.
5. Encourage interdepartmental resource sharing.
6. Develop an in-house training programme.

"Traditional" Library Services

The library is no longer a monopoly supplier of current medical information. Inevitably, this was the area particularly affected by the pressure to contain costs. Subscriptions to many of the library's current journals were ended after surveys showed underuse. Spending on non-historical monographs was also hit. Many sectors of the market were unaffected by this move but there was still a demand for current information. However, staff felt that these cuts need not mean the end of the library's current services and that cost-effective information technology could be used to meet the demand for up-to-date information. This option would also preserve continuity—it was assumed that there was a strong possibility that future medical historians would use computer databases for much of their post-1980 research.

This library was a late user of online services and general information technology—this had its advantages: staff were able to take advantage of cheaper higher-specification PCs and use much more user-friendly communications software. Most library work is done on a 386sx IBM compatible computer running MS-DOS 5 and Windows 3.1. An internal modem in the machine is used to access (through British Telecom's Global Network Services GNS Dialplus) RadioSuisse Datastar, British Library Blaise Line and Blaise Link, and Maxwell Online's BRS. The British Library's online request service Blaise Line Order is used for most interlibrary loan work. BRS is used to download full-text articles from CCML. Windows cardfile is used to record requests.

According to the Council of Europe, one of the main tasks, for at least the next decade, in many European research libraries will be retrospective cataloguing conversion.[4] In 1992, improving the library's ability to disseminate information on its own extensive holdings has become a top priority. Those involved with the library are particularly attracted to the benefits that could be gained by computerising the library's catalogues. Retrospective cataloguing in machine readable form would allow the College to install an online public-access catalogue. If this ambitious project goes ahead, it is probable that a more network-friendly operating system than MS-DOS (e.g., Unix) would be used. Before the proposed library system is specified the advantages/disadvantages of integrating it with other parts of the College will be considered. Choosing, installing, and using Online Public Access Catalogue (OPAC) hardware and software will involve much work and cost much money but this will not be the crucial element in determining the outcome of this major project. Success will hinge on the quality of the conversion of the RCPE catalogues into a machine readable form. This part of the project will involve the most work (a conservative estimate of the size of the monograph collection is 50,000 records). This will also be the most expensive element. Because of the nature of the RCPE library's stock (a stock check will be essential) it is unlikely that an external service bureau could be employed. In-house conversion using (where possible) records derived from external databases would appear to be the best option. The speed and extent of the retroconversion is still to be discussed in detail and will depend on the availability of funding.

Costs

The RCPE has not invested heavily in information technology. Like many organisations, it is difficult for the College to measure what it is getting out of its IT investment. And as IT becomes integral to the College's operation, it becomes increasingly complicated to track the return on its investment. Also, the introduction of new technology has coincided with demand for new services. In some areas it is relatively easy to cost justify IT (e.g., by showing how much manual work is saved by using word processors to produce college minutes). In other areas it is much more difficult to isolate a computer function and show the improvement it has brought (e.g., how do you gauge the benefit of a quick response to a database inquiry?). Staff may find it possible to do their job faster by using a microcomputer and they may find it more satisfying but there is no guarantee that their overall effectiveness improves.

Conclusion

Library managers in the Royal College of Physicians of Edinburgh have the difficult task of balancing the needs and limited resources of their parent body with their wider responsibilities as curators of a historic collection. In the 1980s, this library found itself in an awkward situation. Although regarded as a valuable resource by readers from outside the College, many of the members who actually paid for the library made little use of its services. Those who did, used the current material which, ironically, was cut to save money. Faced with this situation staff have used IT to continue current services in a cost-effective manner. By involving themselves in general college use of IT, they have tried to impress the opinion formers, and hopefully diminish threats to the library's survival.

IT involvement started when (partly by design and partly by accident) library staff began to operate and maintain a computer support desk. Computer support can be regarded as a classic example of what management theorists call a staff function. Many organisations have problems balancing line and staff, and in the RCPE, library staff have often found themselves in that grey area where the divide between the technical and the organisational blurs. Although still unjamming printers and unravelling software/machine incompatibilities, staff have also been drawn into the political process as the integration of IT into the operational framework of the College has effected the distribution of organisational power. M. Warner writes, "if new technology is introduced into firms which do not adopt new structures, then the costs of implementation may be high and the potential benefits diminished."[5]

Library staff have recently been keeping work diaries. The diaries have confirmed that much time is spent helping with general college computing and that some "traditional" library activities have been pushed into second place. The library is now attempting to scale down its college-wide IT involvement before embarking on catalogue automation. This is proving difficult. At present, the workload does not justify the appointment of a full-time systems manager and despite internal training schemes, the organisation is finding it difficult to duplicate the service the library offers.

The past few years can probably be regarded as partially successful. While current services continue, involvement in IT has helped the library for the future. The fact that we are able to consider catalogue automation suggests guarded optimism may be in order. In small organisations with limited funds, library staff are well placed to provide computer support. However, it is difficult to avoid playing a much larger role because of the numerous opportunities offered by IT.

References

1. W. S. Craig, *History of the Royal College of Physicians of Edinburgh* (Oxford: Blackwell Scientific, 1976), 39–70.
2. P. Kotler, *Marketing for Nonprofit Organisations* (USA: Prentice Hall, 1975).
3. R. Smith, "The end of scientific journals?," *British Medical Journal* 304 (1992): 792–93.
4. Council of Europe Working Party on Retrospective Cataloguing Text of Recommendation R(89)11, 19 September 1989, *IFLA Journal* 16 (1990): 29–31.
5. M. Warner, "New Technology, work organisations and industrial relations," *International Journal of Management Science* 12 (1984): 203–10.

Chapter 15.
Multimedia Medical Education Projects at the National Library of Medicine

Michael J. Ackerman
Chief, Educational Technology Branch
Lister Hill National Center for Biomedical Communications
National Library of Medicine

Abstract

The Lister Hill National Center for Biomedical Communications (LHNCBC) serves as the research and development arm of the National Library of Medicine for the purpose of developing methodologies by which the biomedical literature can be made easily available to the healthcare professional. The Lister Hill Center, as it is frequently called, was established by joint resolution of Congress (Public Law 90-456) in 1968, and named in honor of Senator Lister Hill, a long-time proponent of national healthcare and biomedical science issues. The Educational Technology Branch (ETB) together with The Learning Center for Interactive Technology (TLC) represents a long-standing commitment of the LHNCBC to support and develop methods for training healthcare professionals. TLC serves as a showcase for programs which demonstrate the appropriate use of technology to deliver information to health professionals. ETB employees explore the application of appropriate technology to various educational situations, investigating educational uses of microcomputer and optical disc systems, including barcode, multimedia, and hypermedia methodologies.

The Lister Hill National Center for Biomedical Communications

In its first fifteen years of existence, the Lister Hill Center undertook major experimental programs in the use of satellite-based video and audio conferenceing and educational programming. Researchers at the Lister Hill National Center for Biomedical Communications (LHNCBC) realized the importance of computers in information dissemination and provided support for regional health professions computer networks,[1] and prototype computer information systems development, including the prototyping of the National Library of

Medicine's (NLM) MEDLINE™ system. Today, research and development programs at the LHNCBC fall into three major program areas: (1) computer and information science; (2) biomedical image and communications engineering; and (3) educational technology development.

The Educational Technology Program represents a long-standing commitment of the LHNCBC to support and develop methods for training healthcare professionals. Projects have a strong multimedia component, in many cases combining microcomputer technology with videodisc-based images. The program emphasizes intramural and collaborative development and demonstration of the application of educational technologies to health professions education, and liaison to health professions schools and professional societies for field test and evaluation.

The focus for educational technologies at the LHNCBC is the Educational Technology Branch (ETB). This branch conducts research and development in computer- and optical disc-based interactive technology. It identifies and demonstrates interactive technologies and technology applications which meet needs in health science instruction and the delivery of health science information. Branch members explore the application of appropriate technology to various educational situations, investigating educational uses of microcomputer and optical disc systems, including barcode, multimedia, and hypermedia methodologies. ETB serves as a source for information on available educational programs and authoring software. Information on the effectiveness of these technologies on the educational process is also available.

The Learning Center for Interactive Technology

The Learning Center for Interactive Technology (TLC) was opened in March 1985 as the focus of ETB's efforts to provide health science educators with knowledge about interactive educational technologies and as a showcase for programs which demonstrate the appropriate use of technology to deliver information to health professionals. The 1984 Association of American Medical Colleges General Professional Education of the Physician (GPEP) report emphasized the need to effectively exploit new technology in the service of medical education.[2] Staff of TLC address this need by providing visibility to the appropriate application of technology. TLC serves as a "hands-on" laboratory where visitors may be introduced to the wide range of available interactive technology applications or may spend an extended period exploring and comparing applications and the various uses of interactive educational technology in the health sciences.

TLC staff assist visitors in a variety of ways. Individual or small group tutorials are provided depending on the interests, needs, and time commitment of visitors. Tutorials range from general overview of computer-based interactive technology to self-tutorials and hands-on experience with individual systems. Demonstrations can also be provided to illustrate the diversity of available courseware and the alternatives available for courseware design and delivery. Visitors are encouraged to explore various technology alternatives and to study the assumptions underlying courseware design. TLC staff also serve a clearinghouse function by linking persons with common interests, and referring inquiries to those working in the field.

TLC's collection includes representative state-of-the-art microcomputer and optical disc hardware, and educational software including high-quality working prototypes and commercially available products for health science education. TLC's collection is constantly evolving and expanding as the technology changes. Many of the applications feature the use of a mouse, a touch screen, a barcode reader, or even a voice recognition device as the user interface. The use of CD-ROM, videodisc, write-once, and magneto-optical disk for data storage is demonstrated. The videodisc applications include highly realistic patient simulations, hypermedia, visual databases, and expert systems incorporating image banks. One can explore tutoring systems and programs that "repurpose" existing videodiscs. Hypermedia applications, an authoring system database (AuthorBase), and expert system development software are also available.

TLC also has a model interactive technology training facility which uses microcomputers, videodisc and CD-ROM players, video and data projectors, and a custom-built network linking students with each other and with the instructor. The facility is used for hands-on training of health professions in repurposing, authoring systems, and other subjects related to the health professions use and development of interactive technologies.

Multimedia Project of the National Library of Medicine

In an effort to take a sample of TLC into the field, TLC staff developed the Interactive Technology Sampler videodisc which illustrates a wide range of interactive designs and applications by providing brief overviews of twenty interactive programs. All programs involve applications of microcomputer technology, most also involve applications of optical disc technology and all programs are part of the TLC's collection. The disc is designed for use by TLC staff when making presentations and also as a stand-alone program for individual use. Episodes are short, ranging in length from thirty seconds to just over two minutes. Users can interrupt the presentation at any time and return to the menu. These video vignettes provide both a general introduction to interactive technology and a preview of the kinds of programs on display in TLC.

The disc is not only intended to provide information about programs, but also to explore design strategies. It is designed for use in Level I, Level II, or

Level III modes. The disc can be controlled using the hand-controller, barcode reader, two-screen IBM-compatible systems, two-screen Macintosh systems, or InfoWindow-compatible systems.

Over the years, the staff of the LHNCBC has been involved in many exploratory and novel applications of interactive technology to health professions education and medical information dissemination. The earliest videodisc project was The NLM Video Picture List[3] which demonstrated the use of videodisc technology as a visual database and catalogue. The videodisc contains pictures from the NLM History of Medicine collection. This videodisc is a self-contained Level II application. This means that the videodisc player control program is stored on one of the disc's audio tracks. The program is automatically loaded into the microprocessor built into the videodisc player when the disc is put into the player. Interactivity is accomplished by using the keys on the videodisc player's remote keypad.

The MicroAnatomy Video Library[4] takes the concept of the visual database to the next technology level. This system, composed of a videodisc, Human Light Microscopy, of microscopic images and a database of information which describes those images, was developed at NLM in collaboration with Dr. Frank D. Allan of the George Washington University. Over 2,000 microanatomical images located on the videodisc are accessed by the user through the free-text database program running on an attached microcomputer.

For instructional or testing purposes, slide shows of videodisc images can be created. Images can be collected and arranged as "slide" carrousels. Each carrousel is saved as a "show" file. Slide show files can be edited to include descriptive text about each of the images.

Visual Database with Barcode Access demonstrates the use of barcodes for the random selection access of videodisc images and sound. With texts retrofitted with barcodes, or with texts specifically designed to incorporate them, the user has the flexibility of augmenting the information provided by the text as needed. Dr. Ira R. Telford of the Uniformed Services University of the Health Sciences and Dr. Charles Bridgman of the University of California, San Diego,[5] recently published a histology textbook containing no color plates. The legend for each figure contains a barcode keyed to the Human Light Microscopy videodisc. The barcodes control access to the videodisc-based full-color images and motion sequences which augment an otherwise conventional textbook.

The Orthopaedic Videodisc was produced in collaboration with the American Academy of Orthopaedic Surgeons. The disc contains a library of anatomic, magnetic resonance (MRI), and computer tomography (CT) images of the human knee in three planes (sagittal, axial, and coronal) and anatomical images of the arm in cross-section. MRI and CT images of knees from six cases that were scheduled for arthroscopy are also included.

Computer programs are available to control the display of the knee and arm images. These programs will label the images on command by the user and allow the user to compare anatomical and electronic images of the knee in all three planes. A series of test questions is provided to assess the user's mastery of this content area.

The Suicidal Adolescent: Identification, Risk Assessment, and Intervention[6] was developed jointly by NLM and the National Institute of Mental Health. Originally designed for medical students, the program has proven itself to be useful to other professionals—nurses, social workers, school teachers, and guidance counselors—who have regular contact with teenagers. Its purpose is to raise the consciousness level concerning the "hidden" signs of an impending teenage suicide and what to do about it. The computer-controlled videodisc program includes a series of simulations of depressed adolescents. These simulations are used to highlight interview skills development, decision making in gathering information, assessment of suicide risks, and appropriate intervention. The program also explores physicians' attitudes toward suicidal patients, and presents statistics on adolescent suicide and information on diagnosis and treatment of depression. It can be viewed on a one-screen system with a touch-sensitive screen for user interaction or on the more conventional two-screen system using the computer's cursor keys as the response mechanism.

The NLM's Technological Innovations in Medical Education (TIME) project has developed a series of voice-controlled patient management simulations.[7] The project, under the direction of Dr. William Harless, is currently sponsored by the Pharmaceutical Manufacturers' Association.[8] TIME uses voice control and the interactive drama format to infuse a sense of patient empathy into heathcare teaching. Most videodisc-based simulations are intended for individual student use. However, the TIME dramas are intended to be used by faculty in group teaching situations.

The educational strategy employed by the TIME simulation model is comparable to the "grand rounds" tradition in that a patient with a medical problem of particular interest is presented, interviewed, and discussed. In order to use a TIME simulation, the instructor must first "train" the computer to recognize a vocabulary of medical history concepts and technical terms that are relevant to the problems presented in the case. The instructor then acts as spokesperson for the class while students assume the role of attending physician. There are no lists of options or prompts from the computer to influence their decisions. The class can take a medical history, order diagnostic procedures, and make clinical decisions regarding treatment options. Together they determine the course of action and, in doing so, practice making clinical decisions without risk to a live patient.

The interactive drama format is intended to provide both student and instructor with the opportunity to engage in discovery learning. The outcome of a learning episode depends on decisions made during an episode and on a probability algorithm. Even the instructor cannot predict the course of the case. Good clinical decisions and timely interventions increase the probability of a successful outcome but, as in reality, cannot assure it.

AI/RHEUM[9] is an artificial intelligence consultant system in rheumatology intended for the use of practicing physicians not having specialty training in that field. It is being developed under the direction of Dr. Larry Kingsland and is a knowledge base comprised of two major components: a diagnostic consultant system and a patient management consultant system which deals with cases of rheumatoid arthritis. The AI/RHEUM diagnostic model knows of twenty-six rheumatological diseases and reasons from a patient data checklist of 879 elements. In testing with more than 500 carefully studied clinical cases, the systems agreement with a consensus diagnosis of Board-certified rheumatologists is above 90 percent. The management model giving therapy recommendations for patients has been tested with approximately forty cases. Both systems are presently being evaluated in a clinical setting. AI/RHEUM also has Show me! and Tell me more! features. Using Show me! the computer controls an associated videodisc player to access illustrative examples from a video picture library. The Tell me more! feature causes the computer to formulate an appropriate MEDLINE search. Using an attached modem, the search is automatically run and the findings from the current literature displayed.

The Echocardiography Videodisc Encyclopedia, developed by the LHNCBC in conjunction with Dr. C. Carl Jaffe of the Yale University School of Medicine,[10] is a videodisc-based library of echocardiographs. The accompanying program uses a hypermedia environment to teach echocardiographic image interpretation utilizing online text, animated graphics, and digitized sound. This Macintosh-based program illustrates the use of HyperCard as an interactive videodisc authoring tool. It also demonstrates the use of the seamless jump capacity of videodisc technology to create an endless display of a continuously beating heart from less than three seconds of original video images.

Computer-based Curriculum Delivery System in Pathology is a series of ten videodisc-based pathology units developed at LHNCBC under the direction of Dr. James Woods.[11] It is designed for use in the medical school basic pathology curriculum.[12] Each unit consists of a didactic section and self-test study section. The first videodisc in this series was released in 1983 and covered the topics of cellular alterations and adaptations, and cell injury and cell death. Other topics completed by early 1990 were necrosis, thrombosis, embolism and infarction, edema, congestion, and shock, chronic inflammation and wound healing, acute inflammation I: exudates and phagocytosis, acute inflammation II: chemical mediators, neoplasia I: benign and malignant states, and neoplasia II: metastasis and differentiation.

Each videodisc may be used in Level I (non-interactive play only) mode to present single-concept mini-lectures for those users with very little knowledge of the topic. Each is also usable in Level III (computer controlled) mode by users wishing to augment their knowledge through drill-and-practice, self-study, and self-test. Each videodisc is supported in Level III mode by three presentations: a pre-test, a study module, and a post-test.

A new version of the Medical Pathology software was released in 1991. This version uses a relational database system and permits considerable local control of the presentation parameters such as type of hardware, number of questions in each module, and selection of audio tracks (one disc is bilingual). Though NLM furnishes only an MS-DOS version, the program has been ported by one user to the Macintosh computer.

The newest videodisc program developed at The Lister Hill Center is *Cervical Cancer: Success In Sight.* It is part of a joint development project at the National Cancer Institute.[13] The program was developed for health professionals involved in cervical cancer screening including general practice physicians, internists, nurses, and health technicians. Program topics include incidence and mortality data, risk factors, and the screening process. The program utilizes a visual database of cytology slides to identify adequate and inadequate smears, and histology and cytology slides to identify abnormalities. This program was designed specifically for the IBM M-Motion system.

AuthorBase contains information on over eighty authoring products that use microcomputers common to most medical schools. These systems can be used to author both traditional computer-based instruction or hypertext/hypermedia programs. Some support videodisc, digital video interactive, and compact disc interactive platforms. AuthorBase records provide detailed information about each system, such as: amount of working memory needed to use the software; peripheral devices supported; and whether systems have text, graphic, and/or other editors. Costs and terms, branching, record keeping, and other capabilities are given. Most systems are described as either authoring hypertext/hypermedia or traditional computer-based instruction. The latter includes drill and practice, tutorials, and simulations. The ability to incorporate external files or use a built-in authoring language, which increases system flexibility, is indicated. A brief general description provides an overview of the authoring process and information about a system's special features.

References

1. C. S. Tidball, "Health education network," in E. C. DeLand, ed., *Information Technology in Health Science Education* (New York: Plenum Press, 1978), 195–209.
2. "Association of American Medical Colleges Physicians for the Twenty-first Century" (report of the Panel on the General Professional Education of the Physician

and College Preparation for Medicine), *Journal of Medical Education* 59 (1984): 1–208.

3. Video Picture List: Prints and Photographs Collection. National Library of Medicine, History of Medicine Division, Bethesda, MD.

4. MicroAnatomy Visual Library Videodisc and Control Program. Health Sciences Center for Educational Resources, University of Washington, Seattle, WA 98195.

5. Ira R. Telford and Charles C. Bridgman, *Introduction to Functional Histology* (New York: Harper & Row, 1990).

6. The Suicidal Adolescent. National AudioVisual Center, Customer Service Section, Capitol Heights, MD.

7. William G. Harless, "An interactive videodisc drama: the case of Frank Hall," *Journal of Computer-Based Instruction* 13(4)(1986): 113–16.

8. Pharmaceutical Manufacturers' Association Education and Research Institute, Arlington, VA.

9. Lawrence C. Kingsland, Donald A. B. Lindberg, and Gordon C. Sharp, "Anatomy of a knowledge-based consultant system: AI/RHEUM," *MD Computing* 3(5) (1986): 18–26.

10. Department of Diagnostic Imaging, Yale University School of Medicine, New Haven, CT.

11. Educational Technology Branch, National Library of Medicine, Bethesda, MD.

12. James W. Woods et al., "Teaching pathology in the 21st century," *Archives of Pathology and Laboratory Medicine* 112 (1988): 852–56.

13. Early Detection Branch, National Cancer Institute, Bethesda, MD.

CHAPTER 16.
MEDIA: INTEGRATION AND
EVOLUTION IN A MEDICAL CENTER

Malcolm Brantz
Associate Director for the Media/Computer Center
Library and Biomedical Communications Center
Washington University School of Medicine

Susan Crawford
Professor of Biomedical Communication and
Director, Library and Biomedical Communications Center
Washington University School of Medicine

Abstract

The interface of media, computers, and communications technology is an important advancement that has greatly expanded the human capability for information processing. This chapter traces the evolution of the media/computer center at Washington University in three stages. It examines the profound effects on the role of the library and its place in the organization of the medical center. Finally, it suggests projected changes in media and technology that will impact the library.

Introduction

In the late 1950s and early 1960s, biomedical communications as a specialty evolved from the independent activities of medical illustration, graphic design, medical photography, medical television, and audiovisual facilities in libraries.[1] During the 1970s, the focus turned to integration of relationships among these services to develop biomedical communications centers.[2] By 1976, the Association of Biomedical Communications Directors was formed.

Two influential reports in the 1980s subsequently gave impetus to strategic planning of communications systems in medical centers. In 1982, Matheson and Cooper called for the integration of information systems to support research, teaching, patient care, and administration.[3] The 1984 Association of American Medical Colleges General Professional Education of the Physician (GPEP) report, "Physicians for the Twenty-First Century," emphasized general education of the physician and development of independent learning skills that would endure throughout a lifetime.[4] A corollary was modification of learning environments to include the spectrum of media and methods.[5] It was during the late 1980s that the medical informatics movement expanded the field by relating media to human information processing and computer/network technology.

Planning the Media/Computer Center at Washington University

By 1983, Washington University began planning its first new library in seventy years. Early in the conceptualizing, it was decided that there would be two tracks. The library would continue doing what it was presently doing: acquire publications, process and deliver documents, and retrieve information from both electronic and published sources.

It was also anticipated that new resources and technology would interact to supplement and to continually change the present configuration.[6]

Analysis of the institutional environment showed that the School of Medicine was made up of autonomous units that were highly decentralized. Likewise, biomedical communications services were independently administered. There was a Department of Medical Illustration that served the school, but units performing the same functions co-existed in other departments (e.g., surgery). Computer graphics services were provided by a unit under general administration, but functions dovetailed with other departments. Both the Medical Computing Facility and the Biomedical Research Computing Center have educational and research functions. Audiovisual support services (sound and projection presentations) were provided by the library, by several departments, and by commercial organizations. In 1987, biomedical communications services at the medical center could be characterized as isolated, redundant, and disorganized.

Figure 1 shows the information context in which the Library and Biomedical Communications Center presently operates. Through local area networks (LANs), it interfaces with hospital information systems, the medical school administration, biomedical research settings, educational programs, and community healthcare institutions. At the heart is the library's Bibliographic Access and Control System (BACS), an umbrella term for a family of software to access health-related information, ranging from locally mounted databases to CD-ROM and remote databanks such as GenBank. BACS provides a flexible framework for accessing, handling, and networking a variety of information.

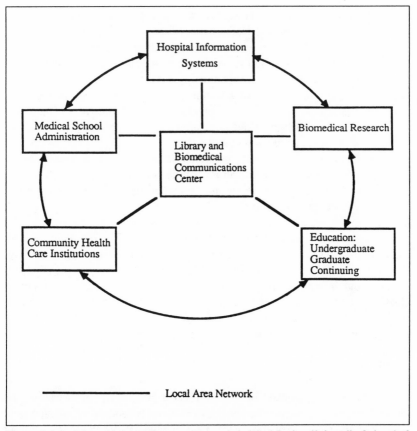

Figure 1. Interface of information components in Washington University School of Medicine Library and Biomedical Communications

The library now manages the network for the medical school's administrative database for financial, personnel, and long-range planning. The Center is also managing access to the genetics database of the National Library of Medicine (NLM) and coordinating its use in the medical center. It is within this context that the library began planning for a new media and computer center which would assume biomedical communications functions.

Goals of the Media/Computer Center

The goal is to apply and to integrate multimedia and information technology in support of research, teaching, patient care, and administration. The present functions of the Media/Computer Center (MCC) are:

- to make information resources available: media, technology, software, networks, databases;
- to provide support services: using hardware and software, virus detection, administering audiovisual media, scanning text and images, managing information;
- to teach application of information technology: group and individual instruction in using computers and software, accessing databases, managing files, and applying new teaching tools and clinical decision-support systems;
- to produce educational programs using facilities of the Center: graphics, videos, publications, similations; and
- to integrate resources and procedures in information technology for the medical center.

As shown in Figure 2, the new media center has 3,333 square feet with forty-eight workstations for learning and for information viewing, accessing, and managing. Some 1,826 square feet house the software and equipment collections and offices for professionals and for support staff. Two modular classrooms, seating a total of approximately one hundred persons, account for 1,972 square feet. There are five group study rooms that accommodate up to eight people each, with provision for use of multimedia.

Information Resources

The MCC developed from the audiovisual library, which focused on the display and use of media. Today, services have broadened to include both media use and technology application. Current media consist primarily of laser disc, videotapes, slides, records, tapes, and other free-standing physical media. New technology include a library of software and personal computers that connect with national and international networks. The interface between media and technology for computer-interactive video, computer-assisted learning, simulation, and other teaching and support services is the direction where the Center is going.

Currently, Macintosh PCs are connected to LANs to provide maximum advantage in using software. The Macintosh PCs also host interactive teaching programs developed by medical school faculty with assistance of the media center staff. MS-DOS computers are equipped with hard drives on which multiple programs have been loaded, and data lines and telephone lines connect them to regional and national networks. Some smaller databases, such as AMA-FRIEDA (for residency programs) and Phase I of the National Board Examination, have been installed on PCs. Larger databases such as MEDLINE and Current Contents, which have been downloaded into the medical center's computers, are accessible from the Center.

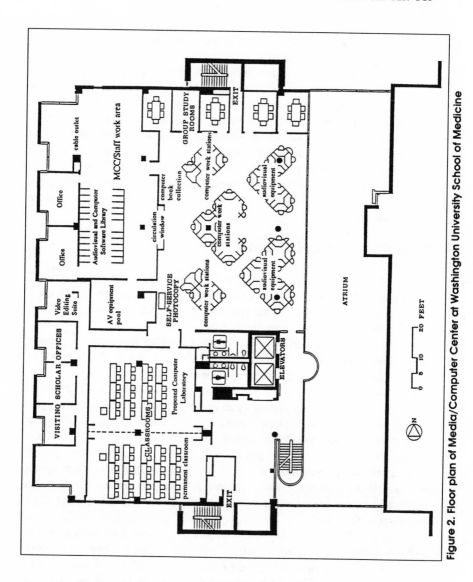

Figure 2. Floor plan of Media/Computer Center at Washington University School of Medicine

Other equipment includes laser and dot-matrix printers, a color scanner for image and text recognition, and a range of software, for example, to demonstrate heart sounds. A computerized book on molecular biology, videodisc players and monitors, and a computer-based teaching program on Alzheimer's disease were recently acquired. The university's broadband network is linked to media center classrooms and to group study rooms. This network broadcasts satellite transmissions of scientific meetings and closed-circuit video. It is also used to televise SCOLA (Satellite Communications for Learning Associated) foreign language news broadcasts.

The library's BACS system provides a window to resources of Washington University's Library and Biomedical Communications Center and departments and hospitals in the medical center. Media, computer software, and equipment in the Center are integrated into the BACS online catalog. A published version of *Audiovisuals Catalog*, which lists resources by broad subject categories, is also distributed within and outside the medical center.

Use of audiovisuals and most equipment in the Center is through self-service with support from the staff for handling and troubleshooting. Computer software manuals and a "core collection" of computer books are among guides to applications.

Educational and Support Services

Because technology changes at such a rapid pace, important functions of the Center are teaching its use and providing support in its use. Presently, seven full-time staff are required to support functions which used to be primarily custodial in nature, but are now highly specialized.

The Center needs to be staffed, during working hours, with computer technicians who make media, technology, and software available and who oversee their use and operation. Daily operations range from routine to complicated, such as, beginning a procedure, repairing breakdowns in equipment, and applying software for statistical analyses. An important program is providing audiovisual (AV) support services for teaching, lectures, and other presentations. Before the Center assumed responsibility, AV support services always ran a deficit of some 25 percent, but in 1991, a profit was finally made over expenses. Services have also been integrated so that faculty can update lectures on a personal computer, reserve AV support services, have slides made, and give a presentation, all within the Library and Biomedical Communications Center.

Several divisions of the library are involved in teaching the use of new technology for accessing and managing information, for graduate and continuing education, and for research and patient care. Teaching by the library staff has been integrated within the curriculum for first-year medical students. The organization of biomedical information and strategies for solving information problems are modules within a course on problem-based learning.

As new teaching tools are developed by the medical center staff and by other institutions, it is the role of the media center to assess needs, to evaluate for acquisition, and to teach their use. Slice of Life, a computer-based laser disc for teaching anatomy, the Human Light Microscopic Anatomy, The Anatomy Project: the Hand, and Cardiovascular Lab I are representative titles.

Present services include:

- producing educational materials: videocassettes, audio recordings, and slide/tape or disc recordings;
- digitizing images for networking and storage (see Figure 3);
- optical character recognition (OCR) scanning to convert both text and images to machine-readable format; and
- conversion of slide format to videocassette format.

A strategic plan to keep abreast of new technology for demonstration, study, and use and to upgrade equipment and resources was prepared in 1991. Subsequently, a $500,000 budget, over a four-year period, was approved which will enable the Center to create an enhanced service and learning environment.

Projections for the Future

The MCC is an important component of the larger communications system of the medical center that includes the computer facility, the library, and the patient care and research information systems. Functionally, it will be increas-

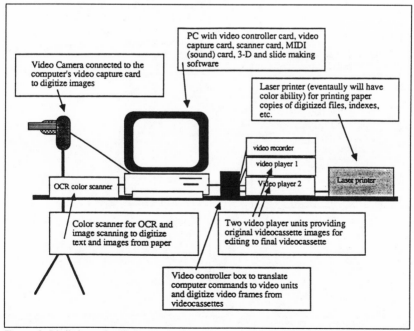

Figure 3. Digital production unit

ingly difficult to separate the MCC from the other components of the system, as they interact to support the teaching, research, and patient care missions of the medical center.

An immediate goal at Washington University is integration of media resources and production into a cost center to consolidate resources and personnel and to assume some independence by generating revenue through services. As shown in Figure 4, networks, multimedia, computer graphics, medical illustration, photography, publishing, and television will become one administrative unit for services/materials production and for instruction/research/evaluation.

Services include providing facilities and assistance for accessing and using multimedia, computer workstations, communications networks, and teaching laboratories. Computer graphics and publishing (both electronic and print) will be handled by the Center. Research support will be provided for the medical center by library staff or through a network of scientists identified by

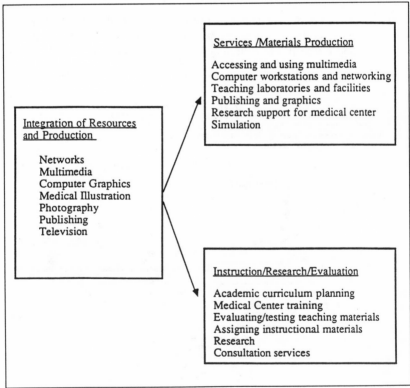

Figure 4. Integration of resources and production of biomedical communications functions

speciality. Instruction/research/evaluation include academic curriculum planning on the undergraduate and graduate levels. Training and technical assistance will be provided for medical center staff. Instructional materials, developed with faculty, will be tested and evaluated. Staff will provide consultation services in materials selection, use, and production.

Long-Range Planning

For long-range planning, the following projections are assumed.

Media applications will be increasingly involved with computers that are linked by high-speed, local and remote networks. Communication is interactive with the infrastructure largely transparent to the user. For teaching, this enables "team learning," distributed classrooms, and networking of multimedia computer-assisted instruction (CAI) to the community. The networks will connect with local and remote databases that merge voice, data, text, and images. Local databases include patient data, laboratory results, radiology images, and data downloaded in library systems. Among remote databases are the large textual bibliographic indexes, abstracts, and full texts; stores of research data as in GenBank (for genome sequencing); and audiovisual media. International and national computer networks such as Internet will bring new capabilities, among them, file transfers, informal communications among scientists, and access to databases in numerous disciplines via personal computer.

Hypertext and hypermedia will become increasingly important in presenting and processing information. Hypertext brings together related ideas and information embedded in linear text, that may be searched through microcomputers. Based on the same methods for identifying, indexing, and searching information, hypermedia link video, audio, graphic, and textual media. Digital imaging, in contrast with an entire document stored as image, converts images, both still and video, into digital data. When combined with computer graphics, imaging will have a major impact on education and medical practice. In radiology, for example, 3-D imaging now supplements traditional methods for viewing images in diagnosis and treatment. The MCC plans to have an important role in providing access to image collections.

A recent article in *Science* described "virtual environments" as computer-generated worlds based on media applications.[7] Media, linked to computers, simulate reality to give scientists a new and vital view of the phenomena they are working with. The visualizations enable scientists, for example, to create protein structures on a screen and to discover how they interact with other molecules. The multimedia laboratory at the Library of Congress includes a "virtual reality system" for teaching diagnostic techniques.[8] Other imaging techniques are aimed at letting scientists visually compare multiple sets of changing data such as observed and calculated levels of ozone.

The term "multimedia" originated at a time when media consisted mostly of stand-alone records in books and journals (print), sound recordings (audio), and images (visual). Today, multimedia refers to the interaction of the entire spectrum of media for simulating reality, storing it, and communicating it. Multimedia extends across the entire biomedical communications system of the medical center.

As indicated earlier, the interface of media, computers, and communications technology has expanded human capabilities for information processing. Called "the third branch in science," computer visualization of images has the potential for extending scientists' thinking by allowing them to view objects in ways never possible before.[9]

Libraries will play an important role in both creating media and managing its use. They will work with scientists to create new ways for visualizing and analyzing data, as in the Human Genome Project; to network multimedia technology for supporting rural healthcare; and to form partnerships with university presses for publishing texts. Undoubtedly, there will be profound effects on the role of the library and on the organization of its units and personnel. The School of Medicine's Media/Computer Center is planning this next stage of evolution.

References

1. G. T. Glickman and W. A. Eicholzer, "Biomedical communications centers—a profile/evaluation instrument study of underlying standards," *Journal of Biomedical Communications* (Winter 1987): 2–9.
2. Glickman and Eicholzer, 3.
3. N. W. Matheson and J.A.D. Cooper, "Academic information in the academic health science center: roles for the library in information management," *Journal of Medical Education* 57 (October 1983): 1–93.
4. "American Association of Medical Colleges: physicians for the twenty-first century," *Journal of Medical Education* 59 (1984): 1–27.
5. F. D. Allan and J. L. Bradford, "An analysis of the GPEP report: implications for biomedical communicators," *Journal of Biomedical Communications* (August 1985): 4–11.
6. S. Crawford and B. Halbrook, "Planning a new library in an age of transition: The Washington University School of Library and Biomedical Communications Center," *Bulletin of the Medical Library Association* 78 (July 1990): 283–92.
7. "Computing in science: the third branch of science debuts," *Science* 256 (April 3, 1992): 44–61.
8. "High-tech information lab debuts at LC," *Library Hotline* 21 (April 1992): 44–61.
9. "High-tech information lab debuts at LC," 44–61.

Chapter 17.
Medical Information Management and Libraries: Development of Educational Software at Georgetown University

Anne Seymour
Assistant Director
Biomedical Information Resources Center
Georgetown University Medical Center
Dahlgren Memorial Library

Naomi C. Broering
Director, Biomedical Information Resources Center
and Medical Center Librarian
Georgetown University Medical Center
Dahlgren Memorial Library

Abstract

The Dahlgren Memorial Library at Georgetown University Medical Center is responding to the need to integrate medical informatics into the curriculum. The Biomedical Information Resources Center (BIRC), a facility for learning, teaching, and development of computer software and systems, was established in the Library in 1986. Librarians and programmers work with medical faculty to develop educational software following several important steps. Five projects are described in this chapter:

1. SuperPATH, computer courseware incorporating digitized pathology slides with text and lecture notes.
2. Microscopic Anatomy Digital Slide Library, a program for studying collections of digitized histology images and accompanying text used in the microanatomy course.
3. Electronic Textbook in Human Physiology, a multimedia learning program covering major concepts in physiology with sound, animations, images, and links to course lecture notes.

4. *History and Physical Writer, an automated patient record system designed for students and residents.*
5. *Fetal Anomalies Teaching Program, a clinical education program for the study of fetal anomalies using digitized radiologic ultrasounds and case histories.*

Introduction

The Georgetown University Medical Center Library is deeply involved with the development of medical educational software. Like many other medical libraries, the Dahlgren Memorial Library is a center for information technology. However, along with managing the learning labs and providing instruction in the use of software, the Library designs and develops educational software to support the medical curriculum.

Computers in Medical Education

It is important to examine the steps towards the development of educational software in order to understand the process and appreciate the role of medical libraries. Why and how did medical librarians become software developers? Two main driving forces were part of the movement towards software development. As frequently noted in the literature, reports from several leading health organizations called for the integration of computer technology in medical education including: "General Professional Education of the Physician" (GPEP) from the American Association of Medical Colleges[1] and "Executive Management of Computer Resources in the Academic Health Center" by the Association of Academic Health Centers.[2] A report from the Medical Library Association, *Challenge to Action*, specifically focused on the role of librarians in introducing change in medical education.[3] Thus, the need for educational software and its integration in the medical school curriculum was well established and the potential for libraries to play an integral part was reported.

The second driving force was the emerging computer expertise of librarians and their role as educators. While the call for new technology in medical schools was occurring, medical librarians were becoming experts in the use of microcomputers. Through online searching and use of microcomputer productivity tools (word processing, spreadsheets, database management software) librarians learned how to set up different hardware systems and software programs. Patrons came to libraries with questions about software packages and recommendations on computer purchases.

In academic health science libraries, faculty approached librarians with questions about the latest and best computer-assisted instruction (CAI) programs. As librarians increased their knowledge and expertise they built up their software collections. The number of business applications and medical software programs expanded and libraries established collection development policies to accommodate these non-print materials. Frequently, these programs could be adapted based on the needs of the particular site (i.e., additional questions and answers added).

In conjunction with collecting software, libraries established facilities for using software and developing courseware. Faculty needed a place to test programs and work with tools for developing their own materials. Students needed a site to use the programs assigned by instructors.

The Biomedical Information Resource Center

In 1986, Dahlgren Memorial Library's Audiovisual Learning Center with its few Apple II and IBM PC computers was transformed into the Biomedical Information Resources Center (BIRC). Today, the BIRC has over seventy-five microcomputers (IBM, Macintosh, and AT&T) and a software collection of over 400 programs. These computer resources as well as other non-print materials are all available to medical center students, faculty and staff for the use and development of medical and general software. In addition, library staff provides technical support to software developers. The BIRC has become a complete software development facility, new applications can be created, tested on students, refined, included in the curriculum, and taught by library staff.

Phases of Software Development

Currently, the Dahlgren Memorial Library is involved in several medical educational software projects.[4,5] Each project has followed certain stages in the development process:

1. identify needs, resources, and new tools;
2. create prototype;
3. select development tools;
4. develop software in a modular approach;
5. integrate into curriculum;
6. develop instructional training/program; and
7. produce updates and new versions.

It is not absolutely necessary to follow these steps in developing educational software; however, this process continues to work at Georgetown.

Identifying needs, resources, and new tools is essential before embarking on a software project. Why develop a package that is not needed or will not be used. Because librarians and computer lab staff are keenly aware of the educational needs of students, the library is a perfect place for determining needs. The resources available for software development cover people, materials, and technology. Faculty and clinicians with an interest in computers and education as well as a needed subject expertise can be identified. Other library and hospital/medical center staff with computer skills have a potential for participating in the project. Materials such as slide libraries, image collections, historical items, test banks, and unique collections can be targeted for conversion into new formats. The final resource to identify is the technology available in the library for software development, including hardware platforms, authoring/ programming tools, and off-the-shelf software. By following the microcomputer industry and its role in education, additional new tools and technology for development can be reviewed and acquired later.

Once an objective for a software project is determined and all the resources identified, then a prototype can be designed. Because Macintosh computers are heavily used at the Georgetown Medical Library, educational programs developed are Macintosh-based. The introduction of HyperCard in 1987 put a user-friendly development tool into the hands of experienced programmers and novice users. It provided a good starting point for many of the hypermedia projects at Georgetown serving as both a prototype program and a platform for final products.

HyperCard is just one of many authoring/development tools for creating educational software. Many reviews and lists of products appear in the literature.[6,7] There are also many publications and journals that target multimedia applications and software development in the educational arena.[8,9,10,11] Depending on the nature of the educational program, other multimedia software and hardware may be needed, such as graphics programs for creating images and animations, and scanners for digitizing slides. Development begins once all the tools are selected, programming staff is chosen, and a prototype is completed.

One characteristic of educational software that is well suited to the nonprogramming developer is its modular structure. Many programs can be completed one section at a time or expanded as the material is available. The entire project does not have to be finished before its release to medical students. For example, test questions can be added gradually to a hypertext program with a self-testing feature and a multimedia program in human anatomy can be developed in modules one body structure at a time.

As emphasized previously, the software must be needed and used to be worth the development effort. The most effective way to get health science students to benefit from the software is to integrate it into the curriculum. If a faculty member teaching a course is involved with a project, then of course the use of the software is easily promoted and assigned for class. In other situations the software must be promoted by library staff and faculty must be encouraged to use it in their courses.

Although many hypermedia programs need little explanation, instructional materials and an educational program are still necessary. Librarians in their functions as educators and technical writers design the teaching programs.

A final step, also an ongoing stage, is the continual refinement of the medical software. Suggestions from students and faculty combined with the growing expertise of the developers will result in better and better versions of the software.

Educational Projects at Georgetown

Georgetown has embarked on several educational projects that follow the key steps outlined above. Supported in part by grant funds from the National Library of Medicine (NLM) and the U.S. Department of Education, the Medical Library has played a crucial role in developing the following educational software: the SuperPATH Project in Pathology, the Microscopic Anatomy Digital Slide Library, the Electronic Textbook in Human Physiology, the History & Physical Writer, and the Fetal Anomalies Teaching Program.

SuperPATH

In 1987, Georgetown introduced PathMAC, an image-based teaching program developed at Cornell University Medical College, in the second-year pathology course. Over the next two years changes were made in hardware and software based on Georgetown's needs, as well as advances in computer technology. In 1989, a new Georgetown version of a hypermedia program for the study of pathology emerged named SuperPATH.

Identify Needs and Resources. The Medical Library and the Department of Pathology identified two subject areas for the development of learning programs: autoimmune diseases and neuropathology. Faculty selected slides and accompanying text materials. The Library provided the programming expertise and computer equipment for scanning the images and developing the software. A small Macintosh Ethernet network including a large fileserver and a few student workstations was installed in the Library.

Prototype, Development Tools, and Modules. The prototype for the SuperPATH program was Cornell's PathMAC program which used videodisc images. Pathology faculty felt that the quality of the analog images stored on videodisc was not equal to the quality of full-color digital images achieved using the Library's Barney Slide Scanner. The initial modules of SuperPATH were created using digitized slides and text in a hypertext authoring system called Guide, and later converted to SuperCard, a HyperCard-like authoring software for the Macintosh. The digitized images are stored on a 600MB file-server easily accessed from the networked workstations.

Integration and Instruction. The SuperPATH modules on autoimmune diseases and central nervous system were introduced in the 1990 spring semester. Availability of the programs as a supplemental study tool was announced in class by faculty and students began to request and use the program. The brief online help function demonstrated the easy point-and-click interface of a Macintosh-based hypermedia program and students required little more instruction to use the program.

Future. Plans to add modules in lymphomas, gene mapping, lung pathology, CPCs (Clinico Pathology Conferences held at the university hospital), and an "interesting case" database are underway. As the Library expanded its Ethernet network, more Macintosh stations were able to connect to the Super-PATH system. Students have requested the capability to print key sections and of course they want more new modules.

Students and faculty have responded favorably to alternative methods for the study of pathology beyond the classroom and textbook. The SuperPATH project has been a learning process for the Library and medical school and helped in the development of more medical education programs.

Microscopic Anatomy Digital Slide Library

Applying expertise gained during the SuperPATH project, the Library was able to create another image-based hypermedia program, the Microanatomy Slide Library. First-year medical students in the microscopic anatomy course are required to study Kodachrome slides and complete a workbook covering twenty topics for the laboratory section of the course. The Library chose to convert the traditional program of over 500 slides and accompanying text and tapes to an interactive computer-based program. Now students can study all twenty topics at one workstation and move around freely within each topic without having to change slide carousels.

Prototype and Development. One of the twenty topics, oral structures, was chosen for a prototype and twenty slides and affiliated text were scanned and digitized. SuperCard was used to develop the structure of the program and the scanned images were refined with Adobe Photoshop and Studio 8 graphics software. Like SuperPATH, the program runs on Macintosh II series computers connected to a central fileserver via Ethernet. As more topics were added (cell biology, ephithelium and glands, connective tissue, and bone development), the program was divided into three major sections: general, identification, and quiz. The general section of each topic includes the majority of the slides with their text while the identification section allows self-assessment by identifying structures pictured in the image with a click of the mouse. The quiz section provides immediate feedback and tabulated results.

The program's typical Macintosh interface allows the user to move from slide to slide, section to section, and topic to topic by pointing and clicking.

Another feature in each topic, the Slide Gallery, enables the student to chose a slide from a menu of thumbnail pictures and be presented with the full image and its notes.

Integration and Instruction. All twenty topics were completed and released to the students on an informal basis during the 1991–92 school year. Students enthusiastically welcomed the new format for studying microscopic anatomy and easily adapted to using the Macintosh computer and the Microanatomy Slide Library program. Word about the program spread as students told their colleagues. Soon, more computers were being used than slide projectors for studying the images. Again, a simple online help function is incorporated in the system explaining how to navigate the software. Students frequently did not even use it. A formal announcement about the program was made at the start of the microanatomy course in the fall of 1992. An influx of students is expected in the Library's Biomedical Information Resources Center as the laboratory begins.

Future. Continuous refinement of the Microanatomy Slide Library program is made as students and faculty provide ongoing corrections in the text, identifications, and orientation of images. The Library needs to work with the anatomy department faculty to fully implement the quiz section. The software was updated so that linking to images on a fileserver can be made at other sites with the software and eventually workstations in other parts of the Medical Center will be connected via Ethernet to the microanatomy program and other image-based educational software.

Electronic Textbook in Human Physiology

The Library approached the chairman of the physiology department about creating an electronic textbook. Supported by a grant from the U.S. Department of Education, these two departments joined efforts to develop a prototype hypermedia program in human physiology. The study of physiology contains many concepts that can be enhanced with animated demonstrations and a non-linear (i.e., hypertext) approach to learning. The Electronic Textbook in Human Physiology goes further into multimedia design than the SuperPATH or microanatomy programs as it also incorporates animations and sound.

Prototype and Development. A rudimentary module of the cardiac cycle was developed for the Macintosh computer using a package called HyperBook based on HyperCard. The program contained animations of electrical and mechanical events of the heart, lecture notes, text, a glossary, illustrations, and sound. As library staff became better versed with multimedia tools, the program was converted to a SuperCard shell, and animations and sound were improved with the use of MacroMind Director and MacRecorder software. Scanned images were later enhanced with Studio 8.

The animations can be viewed in their entirety or can be displayed step by step with integrated text and sound. Among many options, the student is able to study the animated moving heart in detail and the mapped tracking of ventricular pressure and volume. Clicking on a bold word in the text brings up a glossary window with a definition of the term. A multiple-part quiz provides immediate feedback to answers as well as tabulated results. The program runs on a Macintosh II series computer with a color monitor, a minimum of 8MB RAM, and an 80MB hard drive.

Modules. Modular development is especially well suited to the Electronic Textbook. As modules are completed they can be released while work continues on additional modules. Faculty create animations and develop content and the Library's programmer refines the material and incorporates it into the SuperCard structure. The program's integrity is not compromised by this approach since the modules do not rely on each other. Only certain modules need to be installed on certain machines which saves hard drive space.

Currently, the cardiac module is fully complete with all animations, text and the quiz section. Close to completion are the renal and endocrine modules. The nervous system, gastrointestinal, and pulmonary modules are in earlier stages.

Integration and Instruction. Students have been exposed to the program in different ways. In one physiology lecture class the instructor used the program to demonstrate certain cardiac functions. In April 1991, a third of the physiology class used the program in a computer lab session in place of the standard dissection lab. The students were given an online pre- and post-quiz to measure comprehension of the material after using the software. Overall, the students were pleased with the Electronic Textbook and asked for additional modules, especially before exams. Now that more modules are coming close to completion, the program is promoted during the physiology course and students are encouraged to use it for supplemental studying.

The interface to the program is similar to the other hypermedia/multimedia programs with easy navigation plus a few additional features. Online help is available and little formal instruction is needed.

Future. As technology for storage and compression of digital information improves, more and more material can be added to the Electronic Textbook without serious space considerations. Full implementation of linking to the indexed class lecture notes pertinent to each module is under development. New multimedia capabilities are announced everyday. The recent release of Apple's Quicktime, a tool for playing video through the Macintosh, offers exciting possibilities for this and other educational projects.

History & Physical Writer and the MAClinical Workstation

The History and Physical (H&P) Writer is a software program used by students and residents to prepare an automated record on patients they examine. It is one of the many programs installed on the MAClinical Workstations distributed in Georgetown University Hospital conference rooms and resident offices and at affiliated hospitals. The MAClinical Workstation Project was launched in 1987 with the placement of nine Macintosh computers installed with software for physicians-in-training to develop computer skills and experience in medical informatics. The project has now placed over thirty Macintosh II series computers and ImageWriter printers all connected to the IAIMS Knowledge Network of databases. A key element of the project was the development of H&P Writer.

Prototype and Development. The initial version of the software, Hype-Rite-Up, was developed in HyperCard. In 1990, the HyperCard program was converted to C language for speed and development purposes and renamed H&P Writer. The program incorporates a typical Macintosh interface with pull-down menus, pop-up lists, cut-and-paste, and point-and-click functions. With minimal typing users can enter a patient record and print the resulting chart.

There are eight sections to the program: log-in (student information), demographics (patient information), history (including a family tree), review of systems, physical exam, lab tests, procedures and operations, and assessment and plan. Each section has relevant pre-entered lists of commonly used terms, symptoms, medications, or diseases to make data entry easier and to prevent misspellings. Templates and charts for easy entry of lab results, vital signs, and family history are featured.

Library staff also continue to update the other reference software on the workstations and provide instructional and technical support for the MAClinical workstations.

Integration and Instruction. Students are expected to use the H&P Writer at several points during their education at Georgetown. Many medical students use the program to complete patient write-ups in the physical diagnosis course.

Second-year students are required to complete a history and physical report using the software during the medical data and reasoning laboratory. Recently, clinical course directors implemented use of H&P Writer as a required component of third- and fourth-year clinical rotations so they can track the types of patients seen by students.

Instruction takes place in the BIRC or at the MAClinical site in the hospital wards. Librarians provide the instruction and technical support along with a programmer and a technician.

Future Versions. Improvements to the software are often made and lists of terms updated resulting in new versions. New features will include a quick connection to the Library's database for reference, copying of information, and returning to the patient's history and physical report to record the collected information. Also envisioned is a central database for collection of student clinical data via the network.

Fetal Anomalies Teaching Program

The latest project the Library has undertaken is the creation of a hypermedia knowledge base of digitized ultrasound images of fetal anomalies. Over sixty cases with close to two hundred images illustrating fetal anomalies have been selected and scanned. The Library, working closely with the radiology department, has identified important features of each image for best illustration of the particular anomaly. These parts of each image can be highlighted with the click of the mouse. Case histories on each patient and a diagnosis will be incorporated into the program. Eventually a self-assessment mode where residents can verify diagnoses of fetal anomalies will be added.

Most radiology residents have few opportunities to study fetal anomalies. This program will provide a unique teaching tool for the radiology department and even other departments.

Other Projects

The Medical Library is also involved in many other educational software projects under development at Georgetown. Through the Integrated Advanced Information Management System (IAIMS) grant and other support, faculty and departments have been provided with equipment and other resources for the creation of educational projects. Library staff provide assistance in the use of authoring programs and other off-the-shelf software as well as technical support and equipment recommendations. The BIRC is an excellent testing and demonstration facility for new software. Students can use any educational software (both commercial and developed in-house) in the BIRC.

Conclusion

The Georgetown Medical Center Library has experienced success in developing educational software and integrating it into the medical school curriculum. Following the key steps outlined in this chapter and receiving generous grant support has enabled the Library to produce software enthusiastically adopted by faculty and well used by students. The Dahlgren Memorial Library, like other health science libraries, is meeting the demand for software development and the integration of these programs in medical education. Students and faculty at the medical school along with librarians are confronting the future of medical education.

Acknowledgements

The projects described in this chapter are supported in part by National Library of Medicine grant #LM04392-07 and the U.S. Department of Education grant #R197D90034.

References

1. *Physicians for the Twenty-first Century; The GPEP Report* (Washington, D.C.: Association of American Medical Colleges, 1984).
2. T. E. Piemme and M. J. Ball, *Executive Management of Computer Resources in the Academic Health Center: A Staff Report* (Washington, D.C.: Association of Academic Health Centers, 1984).
3. Association of Academic Health Sciences Library Directors, Medical Library Association, Joint Task Force to Develop Guidelines for Academic Health Sciences Libraries, *Challenge to Action: Planning and Evaluation Guides for Academic Health Sciences Libraries* (Chicago: Medical Library Association, 1986).
4. N. C. Broering, "Hypermedia in Medical Education: Accent on Libraries' Role," in *Studies in Multimedia* (Medford, NJ: Learned Information, Inc., 1992).
5. N. C. Broering, "The MAClinical Workstation Project and Georgetown University," *Bulletin of the Medical Library Association* 79 (July 1991): 276–81.
6. C. Locatis et al., *Authoring Systems* (Bethesda, MD: U.S. Department of Health and Human Services, Public Health Service, National Institutes of Health, National Library of Medicine, 1992).
7. "Directory of authoring systems," *Instruction Delivery Systems* 5 (1991):16–23.
8. *Syllabus*, Palo Alto, CA: PUBLIX.
9. *Instruction Delivery Systems*, Warrenton, VA: Communicative Technology Corporation.
10. *T.H.E. Journal*, Tustin, CA: Information Synergy Corporation.
11. *NewMedia*, San Mateo, CA: HyperMedia Communications, Inc.

CHAPTER 18.
COMPUTER TRAINING LABS AND MEDICAL EDUCATION SOFTWARE: AN ACADEMIC MEDICAL LIBRARY'S ROLE IN MEDICAL EDUCATION: A USC CASE STUDY

Janis F. Brown
Associate Director, Educational Resources
Norris Medical Library
University of Southern California

Abstract

An academic medical library has many roles to play in medical education. As one example, the Norris Medical Library at the University of Southern California provides microcomputers and educational software to support the health sciences curricula; word processing, spreadsheets and graphics programs to support student papers, notes, and presentations; and online resources to support information needs. In addition, the Library offers a variety of educational and informational services including formal classes, technical consulting, user group sessions, and newsletters. The Library also provides authoring tools and generic videodisc images to encourage development of courseware. The campus derives many benefits from these services, as does the Library. These new library roles will expand as health sciences schools increasingly turn to electronic forms of instruction requiring more student participation.

Introduction and Background

Academic medical libraries have a long history of incorporating learning resources centers and educational media into their facilities and services. In the 1980s as microcomputers became another educational resource, they also were incorporated into several learning resources centers. Since then, with trends pointing to increasing importance of computers and software in medical education, computers have become dominate components of medical libraries.

Although many academic medical libraries provide computer labs and related services, the Norris Medical Library at the University of Southern California (USC) has been at the forefront of this activity. It serves as an example of the library's increasing role in medical education.

The Norris Medical Library is a medium-sized library located on the health sciences campus of the University of Southern California, which is approximately seven miles from the university's main campus. The primary user population includes students, faculty, and staff from the schools of medicine and pharmacy, and departments of physical therapy, occupational therapy, and physician assistants. Student use is heaviest during the pre-clinical years before students continue their training in teaching hospitals scattered throughout the Los Angeles area. The overall user population on the health sciences campus includes approximately 1,000 faculty, 1,675 students, and 3,000 staff. The library staff of 31.5 full-time employees (FTE) includes 12.68 FTE librarians and 18.80 FTE paraprofessional and clerical assistants. The library building, located in the center of the medical campus, occupies 37,616 square feet of space spread over three floors. The traditional pointers to library size include 45,554 book volumes and 2,596 current journal subscriptions. The media collection includes 2,569 titles of which 230 are computer software programs. The Library, which derives funding from each of the schools it serves, reports directly to the vice president for health affairs, who oversees all the health-related schools.

Facilities

Sixty microcomputers are currently available to library users clustered in different locations in the Library. An Apple IIe, the Library's first public access microcomputer, was added to the Learning Resources Center (LRC) in 1984. By 1985, the Library had been awarded IBM PC equipment and quickly saw the need for more extensive computer facilities. In 1986, the Library completed construction of a computer classroom and lab in an area that had been occupied by book stacks and reading space. The DOS-based microcomputer classroom includes an instructor station and twenty student stations. A video projector attached to the instructor station enhances instruction by providing large-screen, color projections (see Figure 1). The classroom is used only for group instruction, computer-based examinations, and other curriculum-based exercises that are assigned to large groups of students at one time.

The microcomputer lab includes sixteen DOS-stations and five Macintosh stations, as well as two dot-matrix printers and two laser printers. The lab is a fairly typical computer lab setting with the stations in rows, users in close proximity to each other, and dot-matrix printers adding to the noise level (see Figure 2). Computer stations have gradually replaced media equipment in the Library's LRC. The LRC began its computer activities as a location primarily

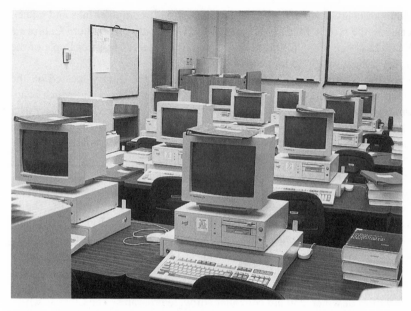

Figure 1. The Norris Medical Library microcomputer classroom includes twenty student stations and one instructor station. A ceiling-mounted video projector connected to the instructor provides high-quality projections for the class instruction. Light switches at the instruction station allow for easy adjustment of the incandescent downlights, flourescent lights, and whiteboard light.

for interactive videodisc stations, but then became the site for other computer equipment as more space was needed. Although still a location for media equipment, today, the LRC includes:

- three DOS-based interactive videodisc stations;
- one Macintosh interactive videodisc station;
- one DOS computer;
- six Macintosh computers; and
- two Unix Sun SPARC computers.

The LRC workstations are installed in carrels providing quieter working space and also room for small groups of students to work through an educational program together. These public access computer facilities also include a desktop scanner with graphics and text-scanning software, disk drives for converting files between Macintosh and DOS formats, and a Macintosh CD-ROM drive.

Adjacent to the reference desk are the four end-user search stations. These DOS-based stations are reserved for searching a ten-year file of MED-LINE and over twelve other databases through the mainframe-based USC

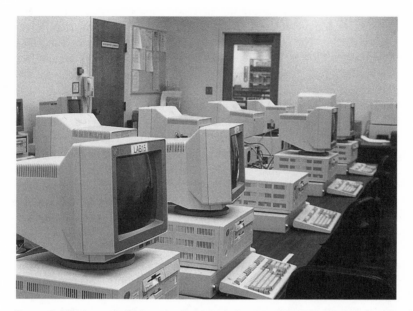

Figure 2. The largest cluster of microcomputers available to users in the Norris Medical Library is located in the microcomputer lab. One of the microcomputer consultants is stationed in the lab during the peak use periods; at other times, a telephone is available for users to call for assistance. Although not visible in this photograph, the lab also includes five Macintosh stations, four dot-matrix printers, and two laser printers.

campus information system, USCInfo, as well as CD-ROM databases. Each of these stations is equipped with an ink-jet printer, though printing from USC-Info is through the Library's high-speed laser printer connected to the university computer network and located at the library loan desk.

Although there are an adequate number of stations for the user population, a few times during the year users need to wait for an available station. Most of the "queuing" occurs with resources that can only be used from one or two stations because of special equipment requirements, such as videodisc players, CD-ROM drives, Macintosh SuperDrives, etc. An annual survey of USC medical students indicates that an increasing number have their own equipment. However, we have not seen a corresponding decrease in use of our facilities. In fact, these "home" users place more demands on the library facilities because they come to the library needing equipment compatible with theirs at home. To keep pace, this has created a need to upgrade our equipment and software continually.

Most of the initial computer equipment was provided through grants from computer manufacturers. Subsequently, however, the Library has replaced the computer equipment to keep up with the changes in technology. In

1990, the IBM PC equipment in the microcomputer classroom was replaced with 386sx stations with VGA monitors through a partial grant from a local computer vendor. The other IBM PC equipment in the LRC was replaced in 1992 with IBM PS/2 57sx stations with VGA monitors through a grant from the university for educational computing facilities. Library revenues were used to cover funding shortfalls.

The Norris Medical Library maintains an Ethernet-based Novell local area network (LAN) to support all the public access computers, as well as approximately forty computers for library staff functions. The network is an integral part of the library facilities and services. The LAN fileserver maintains the majority of the DOS-based software available to users. Although the Macintosh stations are part of the network, only the less frequently used programs are stored on the fileserver. In the LocalTalk-based network, this allows the most commonly used software stored on the individual station hard drives to be more quickly accessed.

Other network services shared among all the public DOS stations are dot-matrix printers, a CD-ROM server, and modems. The LAN also provides access to the university network and the Internet. This allows for connection to:

1. Novell servers in other student labs on campus;
2. the USC campus information system, USCInfo, for searching MEDLINE, PsycLit, the USC online catalog, as well as many other databases; and
3. the myriad of resources available on the Internet.

Generic user identifications (user ids) for USCInfo have been established for each of the public stations, so that all users can gain access to these resources through a menu option with automatic log-on capabilities. Access to other Novell servers and to the Internet resources requires individual userids.

Educational Use of the Software Collection

The primary mission for the public access computer stations is to support the educational and informational needs of the USC health sciences campus. To this end the primary focus for software collection development is educational software and information resources, although other general purpose software is acquired. The software collection includes over 230 titles and has grown rapidly since the first software was purchased in 1984. We are especially interested in interactive video programs and have approximately forty such programs in our collection.

A variety of educational software is available for students. They use tutorials in pharmacology and pathology to study and review material, quizzes in biochemistry to test their understanding of a subject before exams, and inter-active video simulations of patient interviews to develop interviewing skills. Most of the software acquired is intended for independent usage, though some are used for group instruction. For example, HeartLab is used by small groups of students with a faculty mentor in introduction to clinical medicine sessions to learn heart sounds. Cardiovascular Systems and Dynamics, a cardiovascular physiology simulation, is used as a lab exercise for first-year medical students. Most of the educational software is supplemental or optional material, though some are "required" by the faculty (e.g., the National Library of Medicine's pathology interactive video series for second-year medical students).

The Norris Medical Library works very closely with faculty to acquire educational software that is relevant to the curriculum and that accurately re-flects the subject as taught at USC. We diligently collect and scan catalogs, publisher advertisements, conference programs, and journal software reviews. In addition to notifying faculty of available software, the Library also responds to faculty requests for software to be used in courses. Software is previewed by faculty before purchase to determine content accuracy and appropriateness to USC curriculum. We ask faculty for a commitment to use the software be-fore purchasing it, although we do not require assignments to a minimum number of students on an annual basis. Potential usage varies greatly depend-ing on whether the program is intended for an entire medical school class of 136 students or for a small clinical clerkship offered just once per year.

The Library also supports development of educational software by pro-viding courseware authoring tools for faculty. Working with the Department of Medical Education, we have identified authoring programs that are rela-tively easy to use, but which have sufficient power to develop a wide range of courseware. To assist in these efforts, we have acquired as many generic vid-eodiscs as suitable to the medical curriculum such as the Slice of Life, The Atlas of Hematology, Meddix, Human Brain Animations, and others. Very few faculty have been interested in using the authoring software from stations in the library, though there have been several faculty and students who have reviewed the software for possible future use. We experience more use of the generic videodiscs and the interactive programs developed by the faculty. With the Department of Medical Education we have explored the possibility of devel-oping a videodisc from USC images, but until sufficient funding is available or until a sufficient number of digitized images can be stored on a disk, the generic videodiscs seem to be an adequate substitute.

The Library's information services department identifies and selects CD-ROM and other databases that serve user information needs. The Library has worked very closely with the central library system and the university computing services to implement a ten-year file of MEDLINE on the universi-ty's mainframe-based information system, USCInfo. Consequently, the majority of end-user searching is done through USCInfo. The CD-ROM products provide access to other medical databases that are not of sufficient university-wide interest to justify mounting on USCInfo. These include CINAHL, International Pharmaceutical Abstracts, PDQ, Compact Library: AIDS, and Current Contents on Disk. The Library has acquired AMA FREIDA, the microcomputer-based equivalent of the "Green Book," The Directory of Graduate Medical Education Programs, a tool for those applying for medical residencies. However, subscriptions to electronic journals, like The Oniine Journal of Current Clinical Trials, are acquired through the same process as print journals.

Initially, there was some discussion over the appropriateness of including word processing and other office application software in the collection. Nevertheless, they were added because they are tools students need. Students use word processing software for producing research papers and class notes, and they use spreadsheets for collecting and manipulating research data. This was recognized as a way to attract students into the microcomputer facilities where they would become aware of all the software and resources available. Since the library facilities were originally the only (and later the primary) microcomputing facilities on campus, we also felt that it was an important service for students. Incidentally, we face a dilemma of having computers for word processing, but no typewriters. Because the LRC supports graduate programs, we have an extensive collection of statistical software used by the biometry department, as well as faculty and students needing statistics for research projects. We have graphics programs, including the general "paint" programs, and the specific scientific graphing programs which are used for creating presentations and graphics for papers.

The educational resources department decides which office application software to purchase. We usually acquire the "standard" or predominant program for each type of application. For high-use applications, like word processing, we have purchased several different programs to accommodate different user preferences.

Management of Computer Facilities

At the Norris Medical Library, the campus computer lab is a natural extension of our services which capitalizes on our expertise and interests. However, managing these facilities has required a major commitment by the entire library, that includes establishing procedures and policies to deal specifically with computers in the library.

Personnel

The Library is organizationally divided into four areas: information services, technical services, educational resources, and administration. The educational resources department is responsible for supporting the curricula on the health sciences campus and overseeing the microcomputer facilities and the LRC. The department includes two librarians, one who oversees the entire department, and one who works part-time and is primarily responsible for collection development. Two microcomputer consultants provide technical support including (1) user assistance, (2) classroom instruction, (3) LAN management, (4) hardware installation, maintenance, and repair, and (5) software installation. We also have one FTE student position to help the microcomputer consultants provide assistance to users and maintain the facility. A clerical assistant and a .25 FTE student clerical assistant serve as receptionists for the department and provide clerical support. The public computer lab, although partially housed in a separate room, is an integral part of the library and does not require its own staffing to be open to users. During non-peak hours, the facility is open even though there are no computer support staff available to provide assistance. Although maintaining the microcomputer facilities is a major responsibility for the department, it supports the media center, collection development, and provides computer support for library staff and the internal library microcomputer systems.

However, other departments in the library also are involved in the computer facilities and services. The technical services department acquires and catalogs all the computer software. The loan services department provides access to the computers and software. The reference librarians provide instruction, user manuals, and user consultation for the information management products. Providing the microcomputer lab and its various related services requires involvement by almost the entire library.

Budget

The LRC budget includes staff salaries and funds for other operational costs. After staffing, collection development is the major expenditure at the Norris Medical Library. Over the past four years, the Library has spent approximately $18,000 per year in purchasing microcomputer software. An additional $5,000 per year has been spent on information management products including CD-MEDLINE on CD-ROM before it became available through USCInfo. Fortunately, the Library has been able to budget an adequate amount for software during the years we were building the collection. However, as we face times of reduced budgets, the amount available for software and information products may be in jeopardy.

Supplies and repairs also require funding. Approximately $5,000 for supplies is spent annually. Paper, toner cartridges, and ribbons for printing are the primary supplies required. This includes supplies for free dot-matrix printing in the computer lab, ink-jet printing in the end-user areas, and high-speed laser printing for MEDLINE and other USCInfo printouts. However, laser printing in the computer labs for word processing and similar applications is charged at 10 cents per page, to cover the cost of supplies. Approximately $4,000 per year is budgeted for repairs. When the computer lab was first opened, the Library purchased maintenance contracts on the computer equipment. We soon realized we were spending more on the maintenance contracts than we would on repairs. The majority of the problems were those we could repair ourselves, such as faulty disk drives, bad memory chips, etc. We continue to have the Macintosh equipment repaired by outside services, and we continue to maintain a service contract on our LAN fileserver, without which we cannot function and which also was a more expensive system. The repair budget is used for replacement parts, service contracts, and repairs performed by outside services. When we have had funds remaining at the end of the year, we have used them for purchasing small items to upgrade the systems, such as more RAM, faster Ethernet cards, and larger hard drives, for example.

The Norris Medical Library has spent $200,000 to improve the computer facilities. With these funds we have purchased a desktop scanner, videodisc players, monitors, printers, and portions of the LAN including the fileserver, Novell operating system, utilities, wiring, and Ethernet cards. In addition, these funds have been used to replace some of the computer lab computer stations. Even though these one-time funds were available to all departments of the library, the majority were used for computer equipment. This indicates the high priority the computer lab has in the library, as well as the substantial amount of funding required to maintain computer resources.

Policies and Procedures

When the computer lab was initially set up in the mid-1980s, we established many policies and procedures. They were based on existing library policies for other materials and services. Although the Library continues to refine these policies and procedures, they have served us well since they were first instituted.

Only the Library's primary user group has access to the computer facilities; this group is predominantly USC students, faculty, and staff. It also includes staff from the teaching hospitals and clinics. The Library, including the computer facilities, is open to the general public approximately ninety-three hours per week. To monitor access, the power to the computers is controlled by keyed electrical power switches. Only a qualified user can borrow a key from the library's central loan desk to turn on a specific computer station. Controlling use in this way has given us the added benefit of tracking computer use. Users receive the power switch keys in a folder that includes basic policies and instruction sheets for using USCInfo, and peripherals specific to the station, such as the Macintosh CD-ROM drive, the scanner, or the Macintosh

5.25-inch drive or Super Drives for converting files from DOS to Macintosh formats. Use of the Unix Sun SPARC workstations is controlled by user ids which is easier in many respects, but does not provide the same opportunities to track usage.

Users may make reservations to use any of the library's computer stations; however, this is usually only necessary for the high-use stations such as the end-user stations and the Macintosh laser printing stations. Most of the stations are available for two-hour periods, but use can be extended if the station is not in demand by others. The high-use stations have a thirty-minute use period.

The software in the library collection is distributed by three main methods:

1. The majority and high-use software items are installed on the library LAN fileserver.
2. Software circulates on floppy disk through the loan desk, if we are unable to install the software on the LAN.
3. Large storage systems are installed on hard disks at specific stations.

We prefer installing software on the LAN since it provides access from any station, thereby increasing the availability of the software. For similar reasons, we dislike using individual hard drives, which limit accessibility. Use of the end-user stations located near the reference desk is restricted to information resources; however, more experienced searchers who do not need assistance of reference librarians, can access these information resources from other stations in the Library.

For the Macintosh stations we have followed a different procedure for networking software. We install the highest used items on the individual hard drives, since the LocalTalk network does not provide fast enough access to the software. If we were adding the Macintosh stations today, we would rely more on the fileserver and include Ethernet boards and wiring to establish a faster network. Maintaining the individual hard drives becomes an endless job—removing user files and trying to squeeze out more hard disk space to accommodate new versions and new software.

The Library conforms to copyright and licensing agreements. We post warnings about copying software in the computer lab, affix copyright statements to software packaging, only make available the number of copies of a program as we have purchased, and diligently delete all software installed on our hard drives by users. For the LAN, we use metering software such as SaberMeter for the DOS-based software and KeyServer for the Macintosh environment to ensure that only the legitimate number of copies of a software program are in use at one time. We try to keep users from copying software or at least a usable copy. A variety of approaches are used to accomplish this, such as hiding files or making them invisible, only including the files required to run the software and not to install or configure it, etc. There is no data on our success in deterring illegal copying by users.

Protecting against viruses also is an ongoing battle. During the early days of the computer lab we did nothing to protect against viruses, but did not experience any virus "attacks." However, shortly after installing the Macintosh stations, we became aware of the problem, as the Macintosh stations became victims of nvir and other viruses. We did not experience our first virus in the DOS environment until five years after we first made the computer lab available. In recent years viruses in both the DOS and Macintosh environments seem to be rampant on the USC health sciences campus, so we are very diligent in our attempts to keep a virus-free computer lab. We make virus checking software available to users and request that they scan floppy disks before using them in our equipment. However, since we cannot depend on users to do this faithfully, we also have installed RAM-resident virus-checking software, which stops an operation as soon as a virus is detected. Usually this is sufficient to contain virus problems. However, as a back-up measure, the individual station and network hard drives are scanned on a weekly basis or more frequently when we are experiencing a more persistent problem. If this fails and the programs become so infected, we re-install the original software. The LAN file-server has been immune from viruses because we use a program for scanning the network drives to minimize any problems that may occur.

Services and Educational Role

By providing a computer facility, the Library is well positioned to offer other services and to play an even greater educational role. We also manage the computer training facility, which not only provides a facility for our own classes, but also brings us into contact with faculty needing such facilities for their own classes.

The computer facilities are used heavily. Circulation statistics show that the annual computer usage is over 30,000 which accounts for nearly 40 percent of all library circulation. Statistics for applications used on the networked DOS stations shows that the largest percentage of the usage is 40 percent for USCInfo (MEDLINE), 29 percent for word processing, and 9 percent for educational use (see Table 1). Since the opening of the library computer lab, other facilities have been established in the medical and pharmacy schools. Although the students, especially the medical students, use these other computer labs, usage of the library lab has not diminished.

The Norris Medical Library provides workshops on a variety of computer-related topics. A series of ten computer literacy workshops is provided

TABLE 1. Norris Medical Library Microcomputer Use Statistics, 1991-1992

	ref	lab	class	total
Educational Programs	0	1157	229	1386
Information Sources (MEDLINE, other databases, etc.)	3184	2051	515	5750
Word Processing	0	2287	418	2705
Productivity (statistics, spreadsheets, etc.)	0	561	188	749
Other Systems (small, other LANs, etc.)	39	491	124	654
Utilities (disk formatting, file conversion, etc.)	1	39	3	43
TOTAL	**3224**	**6586**	**1477**	**11287**

Utilization of software available from the library's IBM-compatible-based LAN indicating use by function and by location of the use.

ref = end-user station
lab = microcomputer lab station
class = microcomputer classroom station

Total computer utilization including Macintosh and circulated software is 31125 for the same fiscal year.

throughout the year. This includes introductory workshops for the DOS and Macintosh environments, beginning level classes on WordPerfect and Microsoft Word, as well as classes on more advanced topics such as the SAS statistical program, dBase, and electronic mail. The library staff teach most of these two-hour workshops, though staff from other USC departments also participate in instruction. The popularity of these classes has required us to limit enrollment to health sciences campus individuals with priority given to USC students, faculty, and staff, with any remaining openings available to staff from affiliated hospitals. Although the original intention for holding these workshops was to provide instruction to students who are the primary users of the computer lab, the class attendees are more often faculty, staff, medical residents, and fellows.

We have been successful at getting students from each of the schools to attend the introductory training sessions at the beginning of the school year. These usually include a brief introduction to use of the library computer facilities, the basics of microcomputing, and a very short course on word processing—all within approximately two hours! For some of the schools these are mandatory sessions, for others they are voluntary, but usually scheduling these sessions at the very beginning of the school year—or even before school has started—has resulted in good attendance. The immediate goal of these training sessions is to provide the students with sufficient skills to begin using computers for their studies, whether for courseware or word processing. As a long-term goal, we hope their subsequent computer experiences will prepare students for an increasingly automated medical environment.

The Norris Medical Library provides computer literacy training materials that can be used on an individual, as-needed basis. These include computer-based programs, audiocassettes, and videocassettes. We originally felt that the computer-based training programs, such as Learning DOS and the tutorial programs that are included with software such as WordPerfect and Word, were preferable since they required the user to become familiar with computers. However, we found there is more interest in media. Instructional sheets and manuals that we prepared are the most frequently used self-help aids, though these may require human intervention to help users understand the technical instructions.

The reference librarians offer a series of ten information management workshops. They focus primarily on searching USC's campus information system and MEDLINE, though other products covered include CD-ROM systems, GRATEFUL MED, reprint file management, and resources on the Internet. As with the computer literacy series, these classes are taught throughout the year, with special sessions held for specific schools. The medical and pharmacy schools both require students to have MEDLINE training. Medical students receive training during their first year, and pharmacy students receive training during their third and fourth years. The allied health schools, residency programs, and other specialized training programs also schedule the Library to teach MEDLINE to their students. Most of these sessions cover two hours; others involve a lecture followed by hands-on-sessions; a few are a component of other courses in the curriculum that involve assignments that require information-gathering knowledge.

The Norris Medical Library has one of the most far-reaching user training programs among health sciences libraries. In 1991, the Library held 240 sessions with 2,447 attendees. The Library ranked third in the number of attendees at training sessions of the 148 academic health sciences libraries in the

United States and Canada reporting statistics to the Academic Health Sciences Library Directors.[1]

Although not included in our training program statistics, we believe that consulting is another form of training. This one-on-one instruction, though time-intensive, does provide specific instruction when it is needed. To make the best use of limited personnel to support this function, we use a tiered approach to consulting. The student computer consultant is the first level of assistance. The majority of the questions are fairly basic and responses do not require extensive (and more expensive) expertise. We also place limits on our services. Our primary responsibility is to the users in the library computer facilities, although the consultants, including the student assistants, also provide assistance to those who call or come in for advice. However, we refer problems requiring "house calls" to the university computing center. We divide responsibility for USCInfo end-user support—end-users requiring assistance in dialing USCInfo are assisted by the microcomputer consultants; those needing search strategy or database information are assisted by reference librarians.

In addition to a training role, we provide information about computing, especially in a medical environment, to our users. The Library has been sponsoring computer user group meetings for the health sciences campus since the early 1980s, even before we had many computers in the library. The focus of the first meetings were on educational uses of microcomputers. We worked with the Department of Medical Education to promote the use of computers in education by sponsoring meetings featuring demonstrations and descriptions of courseware, authoring tools, and other educational products. For a short time, we expanded this effort by sponsoring additional group meetings on scientific and office applications. Because it later became too difficult and time consuming to separate the overlapping interests, we consolidated our efforts by sponsoring one user group that encompassed all interests. These sessions have developed into seminars on technology topics rather than the typical user group meetings. However, they have been useful sources of information for campus users because they cover a range of topics from demonstrations of clinical problem-solving simulations and imaging software to hardware demonstrations from Apple, IBM, NeXT, and others. The presentations are given by a range of individuals from within the university and from commercial or institutional organizations outside USC. In addition to providing computer information to the campus, we also have used the meetings to generate interest in topics important to the library: using computers for educational and informational purposes. The Library derives many benefits from sponsoring these meetings. Not only do campus users perceive library staff as a source of information about computers, but vendors recognize them as an important group to keep informed about changes, new developments, and special purchase programs.

In addition to the health sciences campus Computer Users Group, the Norris Medical Library also has sponsored meetings of the campus LAN administrators. Although encompassing a much smaller group of individuals on campus, these meetings also have been beneficial. These meetings provide a means for exchanging information among the attendees, including the Library's LAN administrators, as well as hearing presentations on specific topics. In addition, these meetings have kept us in contact with others on campus who are involved in high-end computing and networking, including those responsible for other student computer labs.

The Library's LRC publishes its own bimonthly newsletter to keep campus faculty, staff, and students informed of new software and media programs added to the collection, service changes, and additions to the facilities. Although not an innovative technique, the newsletter is a persistent and effective means of keeping the LRC in the limelight and keeping campus users aware of existing ongoing services and new services. Although we purchase software with a commitment from at least one faculty member who actively participated in the selection process, we increase usage of the programs by publicizing their availability through the newsletter. All new acquisitions are included in the newsletter, which is distributed to all health sciences faculty.

Another service we offer is registering USC health sciences campus users for electronic mail accounts. This service began in 1989 before widespread interest in the Internet was sparked by congressional passage of the National Research and Education Network (NREN) bill in 1991. The increasing attention to the Internet and the information resources available through it will make this service even more important in the future.

As the above examples illustrate, there are many ways that libraries can play roles in the use of computers in medical education, in addition to serving as information resources. They can be involved directly in training students and providing facilities and software for instruction by others. They can promote the use and development of courseware by providing information and resources to faculty. The institution benefits from the Library playing these roles and providing these services. There are also benefits to the Library in terms of its involvement in this area of increasing importance, its increased stature as perceived by others within and outside the institution, its ability to actively participate in the educational process, and its ability to develop partnerships with faculty, university computing personnel, and outside computer vendors.

The Future

We envision continued growth in use of computers on the USC health sciences campus and connections to the university network. This is an opportunity to distribute library services to an increasing user population that does not need to leave their offices or homes to access library resources. We are interested in serving students during their clinical years when they are at remote teaching hospitals throughout the Los Angeles area. There is an increasing interest in multimedia and imaging, and we are looking for efficient and cost-effective ways of providing these services over a network. We also see a growing faculty interest in having students learn information gathering and analyzing skills, so they can continue to learn and acquire knowledge after they leave the university. Our role in this educational process is growing at a rapid pace.

At USC the medical school is moving toward a new curriculum. Although not ready to accept problem-based learning (PBL) for the entire curriculum, the school shows increasing interest in the PBL approach to learning and other means that call for interaction and active student involvement. There are discussions about the importance of acquiring problem-solving skills, life-long learning skills, and information retrieval and analysis skills. Although not a total answer, computer-based education will have an increasingly important role in this new curriculum. This trend is emerging, not just at USC, but in many medical schools throughout the country. This means that on a national scale the role of academic medical libraries in medical education will increase in importance.

Reference

1. *Annual Statistics of Medical School Libraries in the United States and Canada*, 14th No.15 (Houston, TX: Association of Academic Health Sciences Library Directors, 1992), 93.2.

INDEX